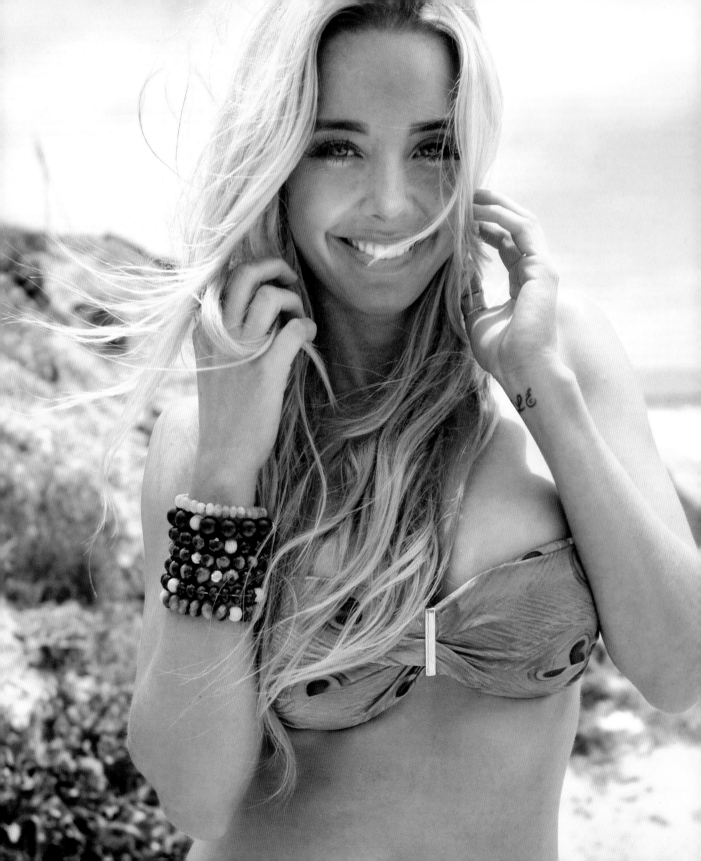

THE SKINNY CONFIDENTIAL™

A BABE'S SEXY, SASSY FITNESS AND LIFESTYLE GUIDE

▲ ▲ ▲

lauryn evarts

creator of the
#1 health and fitness blog,
theskinnyconfidential.com

PAGE STREET
PUBLISHING CO.

PAGE STREET
PUBLISHING CO.

Copyright © 2014 Lauryn Evarts

First published in 2014 by
Page Street Publishing Co.
27 Congress Street, Suite 103
Salem, MA 01970
www.pagestreetpublishing.com

Distributed by Macmillan; sales in Canada by The Canadian Manda Group; distribution in Canada by The Jaguar Book Group.

17   16   15   14   1 2   3   4   5

ISBN-13: 978-1-62414-045-7
ISBN-10: 1-62414-045-9

Library of Congress Control Number: 2013915132

Cover and book design by Page Street Publishing Co.
Photography by Basil Vargas except pages 2, 16, 158 and back cover (top left)
by Sam Blumberg; pages 112, 136, 147, 164, front cover (top left) and back cover
(bottom left) by Katherine Rose; and pages 72, 80, 82, front cover (third left)
by Sandy Spears

Printed and bound in China

Page Street is proud to be a member of 1% for the Planet. Members donate one percent of their sales to one or more of the over 1,500 environmental and sustainability charities across the globe who participate in this program.

TO MY SWEET MOM, WHO TAUGHT ME
HOW TO WORK MY FREAKING ASS OFF

———————————————

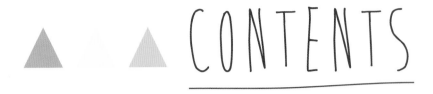

CONTENTS

IT'S A LIFESTYLE, NOT A DIET

Hey, hey!

Welcome to The Skinny Confidential lifestyle.

If you're hoping for a blueprint on how to diet, you're reading the wrong book.

Throughout these pages you won't learn how to deprive yourself.

Diets are deceiving. At first they work swimmingly, but after a while, they catch up to you (and your ass).

The Skinny Confidential lifestyle is about balance, balance, balance and, ultimately, discovering a way to live a healthy, happy life.

Without the deprivation part.

I hope that after reading this book, you'll have learned some tricks of the trade; have discovered healthy, easy recipes; and will recognize the importance of balance.

ULTIMATELY, MY GOALS ARE TO:

+ Change your relationship with exercise. I hope that you'll compare exercise to brushing your teeth—it's something you just do. Not a chore, but a healthy habit.
+ Introduce you to your new bestie: green juice.
+ Demonstrate how ignorance is definitely not bliss. Know what the hell you're putting into your mouth.
+ And lastly, highlight the fact that living a healthy and happy life doesn't need to be so hard.

Balance is key, babes.

Because let's face it: We all want to have our cake and eat it, too!

xx,

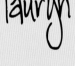

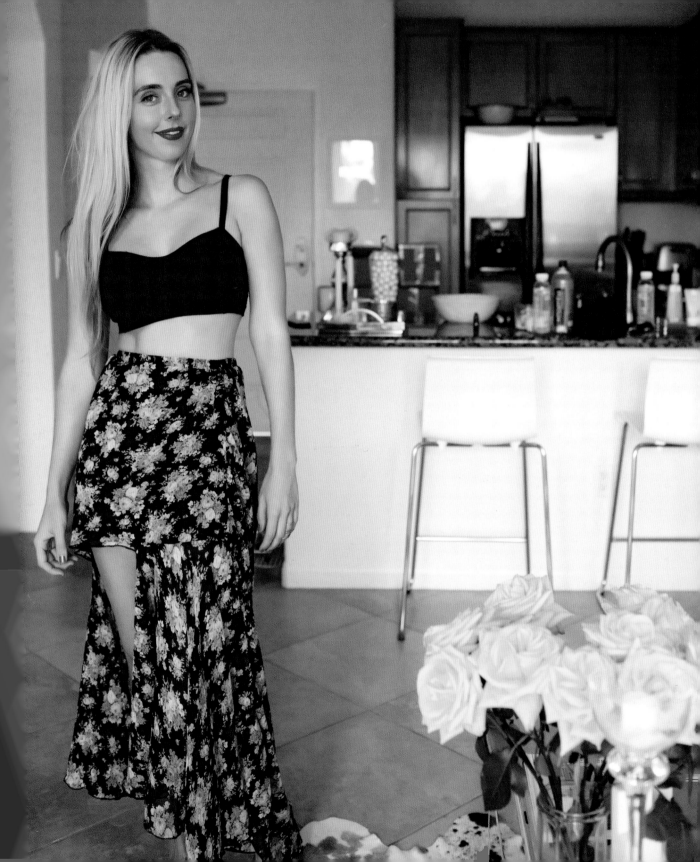

1

FAKE IT
UNTIL YOU MAKE IT

How many times have you heard the phrase, "fake it until you make it"?

I'm guessing a mil?

But have you put it into action?

Really, seriously, honestly ask yourself that question.

SERIOUSLY, SERIOUS?

So, you're feeling overweight and negative. Why not change your attitude? Start by radiating positivity.

If you don't feel positive, fake it.

When you project that energy into the universe, crazy things happen.

The sooner you start living and adopting a healthy, happy lifestyle, the sooner you'll get want you want.

We all have moments of insecurity, but faking confidence is what builds confidence. In many ways, it's a serious ability to be able to walk into a room and pretend like you know what the hell you're doing, when in reality you're completely clueless.

But practice makes perfect.

As with any skill, it takes work. So start practicing confidence. Confidence with your body image. Confidence in your job. Confidence in any relationship.

CONFIDENCE IN LIFE.

It's the key to a happy life. When you feel confident, you feel powerful. Tap into that confidence to achieve the body you've always wanted, the relationship you've always dreamed of, and/or the happy life you've always envisioned for yourself and for those important to you.

If you're eating like shit, you're not confident. You're probably feeling crappy because when you eat like shit, you feel like shit. Start eating healthful foods with confidence.

That's faking it until you make it.

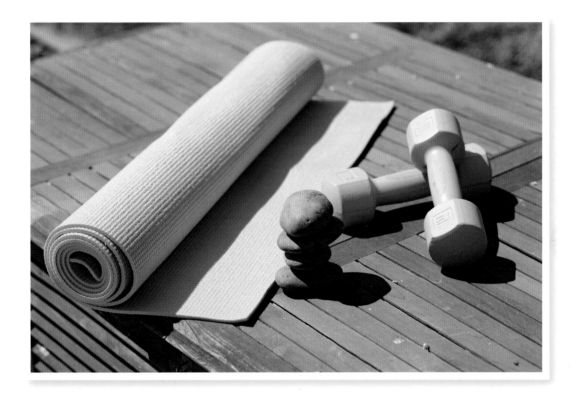

If you want to get on an exercise plan, but you've never pulled the trigger, practice your new skill: confidence.

Start walking for ten minutes a day and add in weights a couple times a week. Fake your workout. Fake like you know what you're doing. With time and a little bit of discipline, you could discover that maybe, actually, you really like breaking a light sweat.

And then you're not faking it; you're loving it.

A relationship you're painfully insecure in? Make a decision. If you decide to continue the relationship, then know with confidence that you're the one who decided to put yourself in the situation. Therefore, it's up to you to be a confident mate.

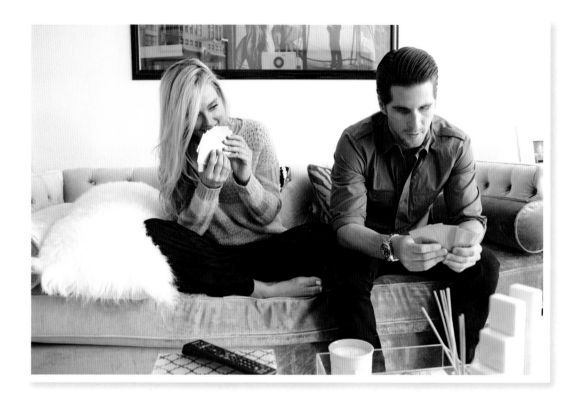

And trust me; any partner is attracted to confidence.

With confidence comes happiness. Faking it until you make it is not necessarily being a fake person. It's changing the tone of your life.

I'll give you an example. My best friend wasn't a big reader. I told her to fake it.

She was obviously confused. What did I mean by "fake" reading?

Welp, I meant fake that you like to read.

So I gave her an easy, quick read. She read it. Slowly. But she finished the entire book.

From there, I had her progress to another quick read that was a bit longer.

She faked liking to read for about three books.

After her third book, she was hooked.

When she went out of her comfort zone, she realized she actually did like reading and was very good at it.

So good that my bestie now calls me with book recs. She's unstoppable.

The point is that sometimes when you fake something, you'll realize that you're actually quite good at it.

If you're an unhealthy person, start faking that you're a healthy person. Do the opposite of all your horribly unhealthy habits.

AND START TODAY. NOT TOMORROW. TODAY.

You just might find you actually like feeling amazing through exercise and diet.

I hope this book encourages you to step out of your comfort zone. I hope it encourages you to be confident, eat clean and sweat often.

Be the best version of you. Even if you have to fake it for a while.

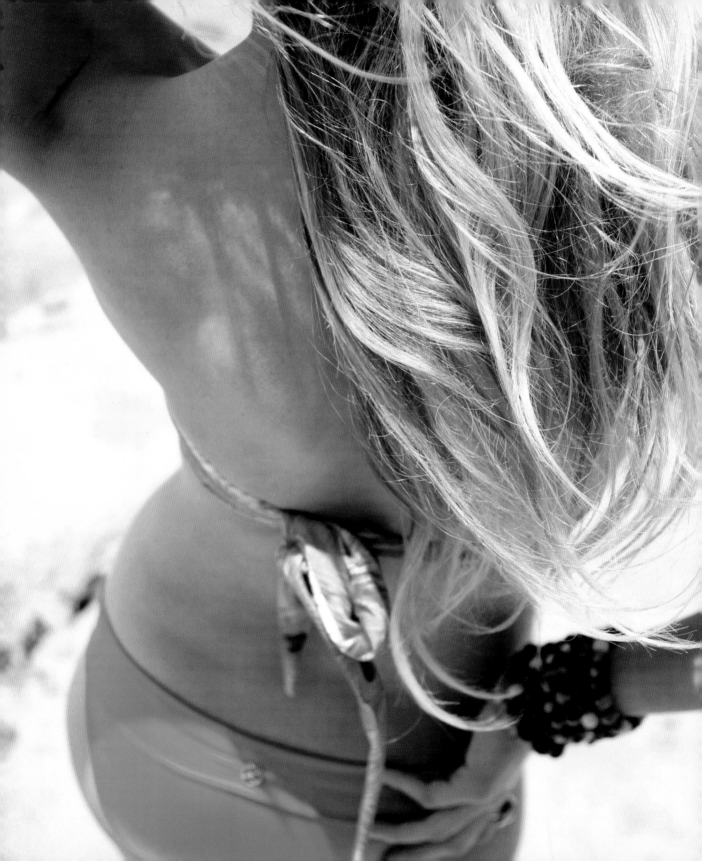

2

CRAVINGS,
SCHMAVINGS

Cravings are like assholes. Everyone has one.

Or ten.

Because show me someone who DOESN'T crave a good handful of Cheez-It®?!

LIKE, REALLY?

In any case, I'm not going to sit here and tell you that The Skinny Confidential lifestyle doesn't allow cravings.

I'm also not going to sit here and tell you that cravings are the devil and you should ignore them at all costs.

And I'm sure as hell not going to tell you to count your calories like they're dollar bills.

If you have a freaking craving, then have a small portion and move on with your life.

Here's the deal: If you obsess over anything (this includes men, too), it will bite you in the ass.

On that note, I guess I'll share my Flamin' Hot Cheetos® story. But don't judge.

One day a few months ago, I had the brilliant idea to stay the F away from the red, MSG-filled little shits that turn anyone's fingers bright red.

But not just for a day. Not just for a month.

FOREVER.

I wanted to nip my awful craving in the bud, ya know?

Because for some reason, that's just what I crave. I can't help it.

Not chocolate-filled cookies.

Not salty-ass crackers.

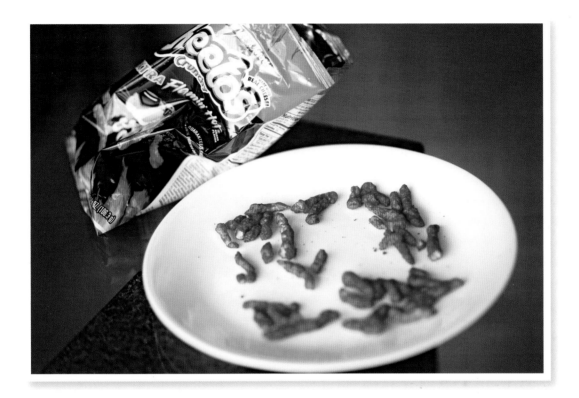

And not even white bread.

Flamin'. Hot. Cheetos®.

They're just really freaking delicious. And they're so bad for you that it's almost embarrassing that I'm putting this horrendous food weakness into writing.

I'm telling ya, though, these overly salted, chemical sticks are truly addictive.

Like, seriously, balls-to-the-walls, can't-get-enough addictive.

I know, I know. Stop shaking your head in disgust, because I've done my research. And I know I might as well take a puff of a cig every time I eat a handful of Cheetos®.

So, weakness admitted. Now back to my brilliant idea: cutting out Cheetos®.

When I decided to ban Cheetos® like they were against my religion, I noticed I craved them even more.

SHOCKER.

Anything, and I mean *anything* that you ban from your life for good, you'll crave more.

My Cheetos® addiction was gnarly. After cutting them out, I noticed my upper lip was sweating and perspiring.

Not really, but you get the gist.

I was freaking seething for Flamin' Hots. I would have done creepy things to get my hands on a bag of those chemicals.

After one month of going Cheeto-less, I caved.

Sadly, I ate an entire bag like they were going out of style. In like, five seconds.

Gross?

I know (shaking my head).

BUT. You know what this little experience taught me?

EVERYTHING IN MODERATION.

I can't stress it enough.

Seriously.

It's simply not necessary (nor does it agree with my normally healthy lifestyle) to shove Cheetos® in my face every day.

But every once in a while?

HELL YA.

Here's what I do now: I eat those red little dipshits when I'm having a craving (about two times a week) and I don't take the bag to bed with me.

Every, single, time I consume something that maybe isn't super healthful, I use portion-controlled kitchenware.

Because that, my friends, is called a lifestyle change. Not a diet. Not deprivation. A solution.

A solution to a situation that will spiral out of control if it becomes unmanageable.

When you deny a strong craving, that's exactly what you're doing, peeps.

You're fighting the inevitable craving.

Fix the problem before it gets super creepy. If you're dying for a banana split, go eat a freaking banana split.

But please, oh, please, practice portion control with each and every craving.

More about portion control:

I'm starting to notice that people would prefer to not really, actually know about true portion control.

Ignorance is not bliss.

KNOW YOUR FACTS!

Because portions are funny.

They sneak up on you if you're not careful.

Check out the portion control chart on the next page. Tattoo this onto your hand and/or memorize it.

As you can see, if you constantly overdo portions, it will sure as hell catch up to you—and your ass.

THE DEETS ON
PORTION
CONTROL

RECOMMENDED PORTIONS PER MEAL

VEGETABLES
UNLIMITED

CARBS
1-2 OZ

PROTEIN
4-6 OZ

EQUIVALENT	FOODS	CALORIES
FIST = 1 CUP	QUINOA / PASTA / FRUIT & VEGGIES	200 / 75 / 40
PALM = 3 OUNCES	MEAT / FISH / POULTRY	160 / 160 / 160
HANDFUL = 1 OUNCE	NUTS / BERRIES	170 / 85
2 HANDFULS = 1 OUNCE	CHIPS / POPCORN / CRACKERS	150 / 120 / 100
THUMB = 1 OUNCE	ALMOND BUTTER / CHEESE	170 / 100
THUMB TIP = 1 OUNCE	COOKING OIL / BUTTER / SUGAR	40 / 35 / 15

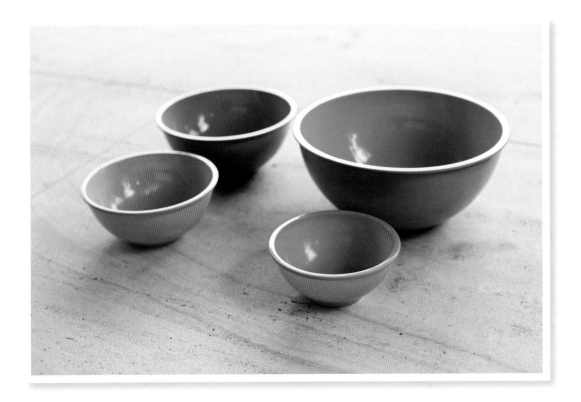

My biggest tip? I don't keep huge plates, bowls or cups in my house.

YUP, YUP, YUP.

All my kitchenware is premeasured to the appropriate portions.

It just makes life easier.

I don't have time to weigh out my meals (I mean, who does?). So having a preportioned bowl in arm's reach keeps me accountable.

Don't cheat yourself. Know how much you're eating.

Life's too short to obsess over foods in a negative way. Make food secondary, not primary.

BTW: You're going to slip up every once in a while, but the cleaner you eat, the better it will be when you do slip up. Eat clean as much as possible, and give in to your cravings in a smart way. Discipline's important, just like with anything else.

The point: If you're really craving something, and you're craving it so badly that after you've eaten a full meal you're still dying for it, then eat it.

But do yourself a favor and eat it in a portion-controlled bowl.

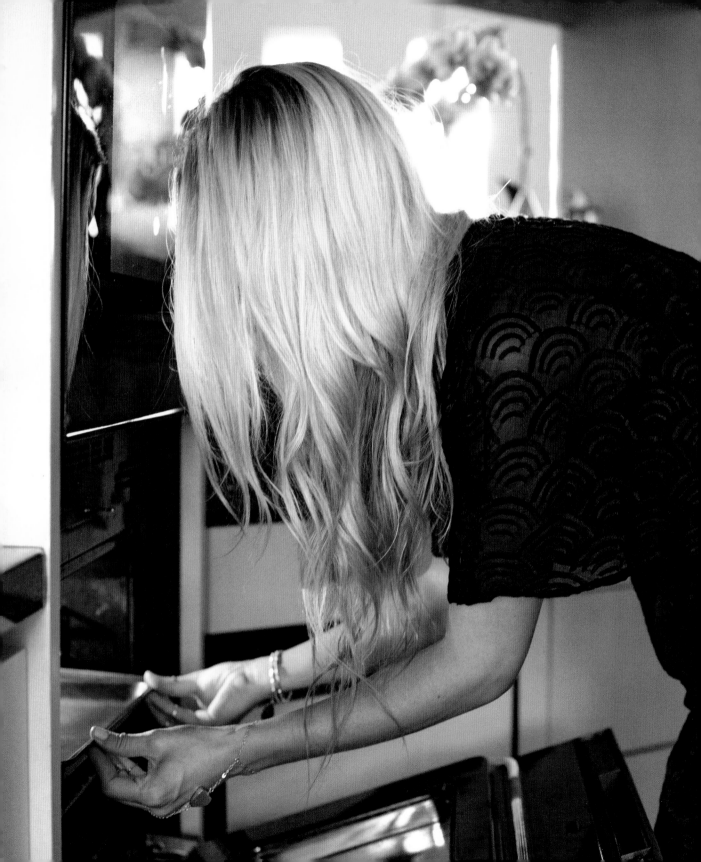

3

SKINNY RECIPES

THAT WILL CHANGE YOUR FREAKING LIFE

Eating healthy doesn't have to be some calorie-counting, crazy diet. The more you fuel your body with healthful foods, the better you'll feel and the better you'll look.

I hate when dietitians tell people to count calories. As if we all don't have enough going on.

I MEAN, RIGHT?!

Geez. I don't have time to sit down and write down every single thing I've eaten every day, plus add up the cals.

Let me give you an easier, more effective alternative that's worked wonders for me: Eat clean. Smaller portions. All in moderation. Make healthy eating and exercise a lifestyle, not a diet.

It's really not rocket science. Choose clean eats over chemicals.

For instance, if given the choice, always pick the all-natural, organic version.

But wait, what about products labeled "diet," "low-fat" or "100 calorie"?

Welp, sorry to burst your bubble: They're nasty. Diet foods are typically filled with artificial sweeteners, lack essential nutrients and don't help fight off diseases.

Eat the real deal: fresh, real foods.

Replace your diet foods with real foods and thank me later.

Think berries, sweet potatoes, seaweeds, salmon, every vegetable, super foods.

SOME OF MY FAVORITE SUPER FOODS:

+ Apples
+ Beans
+ Dark chocolate
+ Eggs
+ Garlic
+ Grapes
+ Green tea
+ Hot peppers
+ Kale
+ Lentils
+ Mushrooms
+ Nuts

+ Olive oil
+ Peaches
+ Pineapples
+ Pomegranates
+ Pumpkin
+ Quinoa
+ Spirulina
+ Sweet potatoes
+ Swiss chard
+ Watermelon
+ Wheat germ
+ Wild-caught salmon

Before I share my staple recipes, let me provide a disclaimer.

I'm not freaking Mario Batali. These measurements are not exact to the decimal. What I can promise is that they're clean recipes—so clean, they don't really need to be exact.

I'm not using flour, sugar or tons of salt—all of which require strict measurements.

For my recipes, if you want to add some more fruit or veggies or an extra egg, go for it.

If you're eating clean, do whatever floats your boat.

SO.

Here's a bunch of simple, easy recipes that aren't exact to the T, but they're all filled with delicious health benefits and will keep you full for a long-ass time.

>BREAKY
A SEX KITTEN'S SALAD

Yes, a salad for breakfast. Weird? Just wait.

This is a fruit salad that will rock your world. It will set the tone for your day and give you sustainable energy. Enjoy this baby with a cup of green tea and you're ready to start the A.M. off right.

SERVES 1

1 handful of strawberries, sliced

1 handful of blueberries

4 hefty pineapple wedges, chopped

1 kiwi, skinned and diced

4 tbsp/30 g Greek yogurt

2 tbsp/20 g chia seeds

Cinnamon, to taste

Pumpkin pie spice, to taste

Nutmeg, to taste

Optional: fresh mint leaves

+ Combine all ingredients in a large bowl and toss lightly. Add extra spices on top. Garnish with mint (optional).

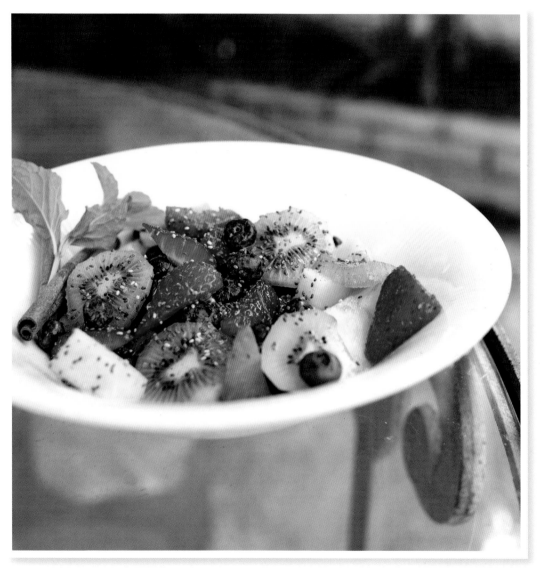

^ A SEX KITTEN'S SALAD

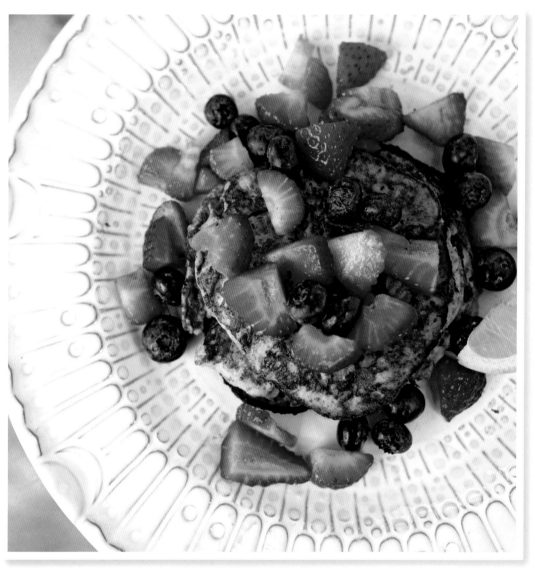

∧ TWO-INGREDIENT PANCAKES

TWO-INGREDIENT PANCAKES

Let me introduce you to heaven on earth: two-ingredient pancakes. This recipe will change your Sunday mornings. Not only will you not feel bloated after a huge breakfast, but you'll feel full, satisfied and healthy!

SERVES: 1-2

½ cup/120 g ripe banana, very mashed
2 eggs
1 heaping tbsp/10 g flaxseed (optional)
Coconut oil cooking spray
Optional: pumpkin spice, cinnamon, berries and a few squeezes of lemon juice

+ Mix banana and eggs in a bowl. Add 1 heaping tbsp/10 g of flaxseed if you want your pancakes to really hold together well. Heat a skillet to medium heat and spray with coconut oil cooking spray. Scoop a bit of batter (think the size of a tennis ball for one pancake) onto the skillet. Cook until the edges are dry. You want your pancake thin. Flip. Cook till golden brown. Goal: 4 to 6 pancakes. I like to add about 3 dashes of pumpkin pie spice. Garnish with a dash of cinnamon, a few berries and a squeeze of lemon.

NOTE: If you're pressed for time, use a blender to mix ingredients.

A VERY VEGGIE SCRAMBLE

This veggie scramble is quick, easy and probably the best breakfast ever because it's full of protein. It will keep your metabolism at an optimal speed, too, because it's full of avocado and veggies. Enjoy this with a cup of green tea and you're golden!

SERVES 1 TO 2

1 white or red onion, chopped

A bit of coconut oil

2 eggs (none of that egg white shit here)

1 handful of arugula

½ tomato, diced

1 avocado, sliced

Optional: a side of pico de gallo or salsa verde

+ Sauté chopped onions in a little bit of coconut oil in a pan on low heat for 1 to 3 minutes. Beat the eggs with a fork or wire whisk. After a few minutes, pour eggs into the pan. While eggs are cooking, arrange a bed of arugula on a plate. Toss the tomatoes and avo slices on top of the lettuce. After the eggs are cooked to your liking, put them on top of your veggie medley. For a condiment, try pico de gallo or salsa verde.

NOTE: The reason I'm not a fan of cooking all the veggies into the eggs is that when you heat vegetables, they lose their nutrients. If you cook the eggs and then add the raw veg, you'll receive more healthy benefits. Also, if you want to add turkey or chicken (extra protein!!) to this scramble, go for it!

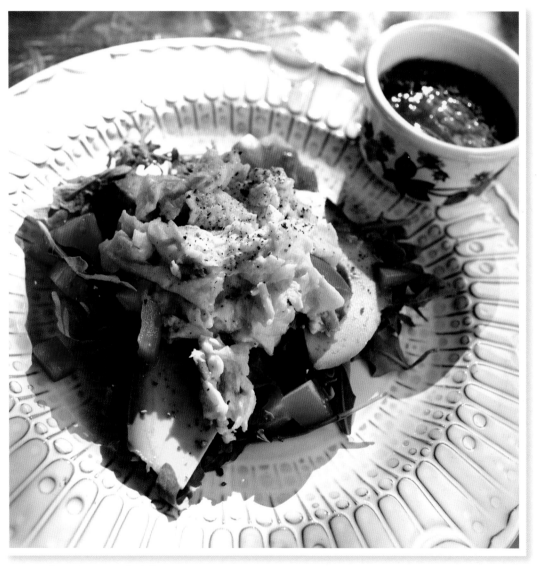

^ A VERY VEGGIE SCRAMBLE

>LUNCH

THE HOLY KALE

Ahhh, kale. If kale were a boy, I'd be crushin'! Kale's is so cool and versatile. My favorite way to eat kale is in a salad. I die over it because it's so filling! This is my favorite salad.

SERVES 2

2 ½ heaping handfuls of kale, chopped

1 handful of baby arugula, washed

1 tangerine, peeled and sectioned

1 tomato, sliced

1 cup/100 g purple or white cauliflower, diced

⅓ cup/70 g scallions, chopped

½ avocado, diced

DRESSING
2 tbsp/10 g Dijon mustard

1 to 2 tbsp/15 to 30 ml of extra virgin olive oil

½ lemon

Sea salt, to taste

Black pepper, to taste

Rosemary or basil, chopped

+ For the salad, combine kale, arugula, tangerine, tomato, cauliflower, scallions and avocado in a large bowl.

For the dressing, mix all ingredients together. Don't think I'm weird, but I like to shake my dressing up in a martini shaker (sans ice, obvi).

Toss salad with the dressing. Add a stick of rosemary or a few leaves of basil for garnish.

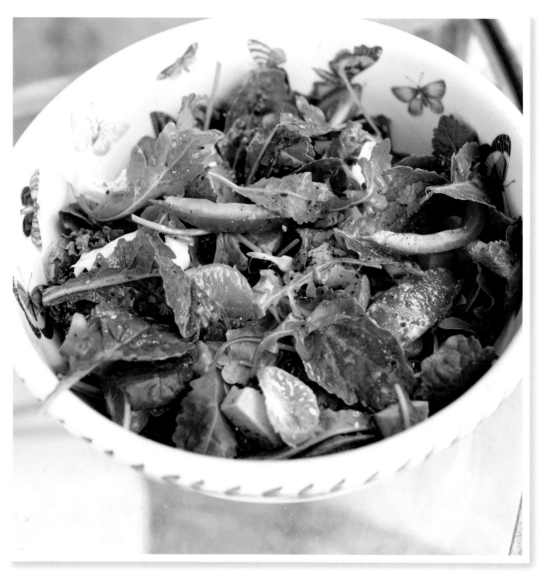

∧ THE HOLY KALE

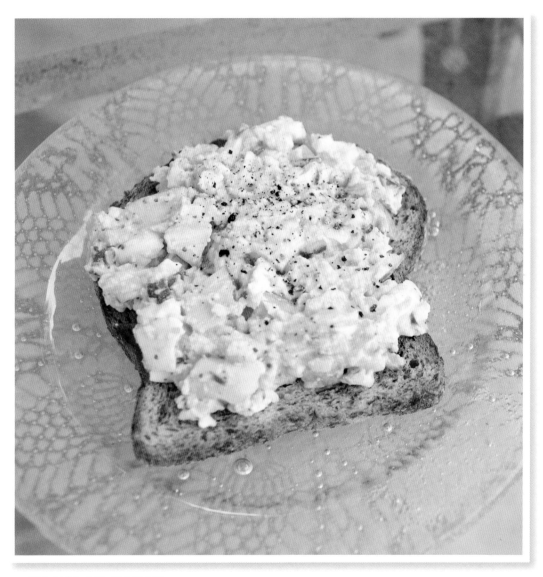

^ THE HALF-ASS SANDWICH

THE HALF-ASS SANDWICH

My grandma makes this little gem for me at least once a month. It's super easy to throw together and works great for lunch (or linner . . . lunch and dinner together).

SERVES 1

3 hard-boiled eggs

2 tbsp/10 g Dijon mustard

1 tbsp/10 g olive oil mayonnaise

6 cornichons, diced

¼ apple, diced

1 slice of low-carb, no-salt bread, toasted

A few dashes of black pepper

A few sprinkles of sea salt

A few dashes of chili flakes, to taste

+ Peel shells off the hard-boiled eggs. Put the shell-less eggs in a large bowl and mash them with a fork. Add Dijon mustard, mayo, cornichons and apple. Add about 3 hefty spoonfuls of the low-cal egg salad onto one (only one! Remember, open-faced) piece of toast. Add pepper, sea salt and chili flakes.

If you have leftover egg salad, don't freak out. Save it for tomorrow. There's no reason to lick the bowl.

SKINNY HOMEMADE LENTIL SOUP

Lentils are seriously insane. Why? Glad you asked.

They're filled with B vitamins, contain tons of fiber and are super filling (hello, protein!). They're also known to help reduce women's risk of developing breast cancer. Gotta protect the girls! Enjoy this recipe, which I stole from my friend Mike because it's too delicious not to share!

SERVES 3 TO 4

2 cups/460 g carrots, chopped

2 cups/460 g celery, chopped

1 large yellow onion, chopped

1 tsp/5 ml coconut cooking oil

24 oz/700 ml vegetable or chicken stock

1 small package dry vegetable/mushroom soup mix, such as Manischewitz®

1 cup/160 g precooked lentils

Sea salt, to taste

Black pepper, to taste

+ In a large saucepan or Dutch oven, sauté the classic trio—carrots, celery and onion—over medium-high heat in the coconut oil. Add the stock and bring to a low boil. Add the dry soup mix (reserve the seasoning pack), return to boil, cover and simmer, as directed by the package, on low heat for 1 ½ hours.

If you're using canned lentils, give them a decent rinse. I've found the precooked packaged ones are perfect, but a little hard to find.

Now, combine the lentils and the seasoning package, add to the soup and simmer another 30 minutes. Season to taste with sea salt and pepper. Let stand and serve.

This recipe evolves with practice. Last time I made it, I added fresh mushrooms and a few splashes of white wine. See what's left in the fridge and have fun.

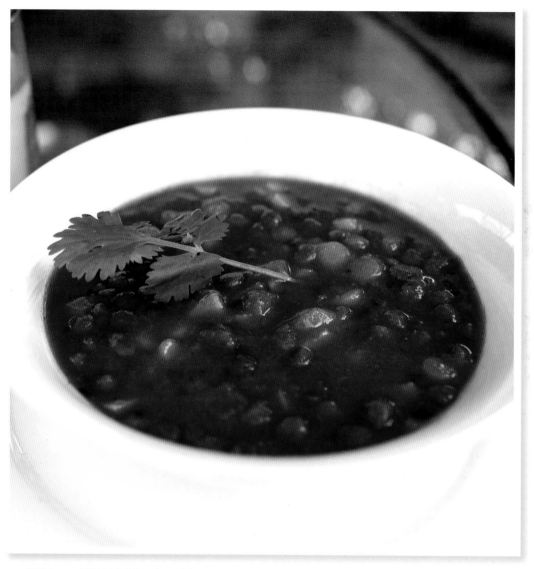

^ SKINNY HOMEMADE LENTIL SOUP

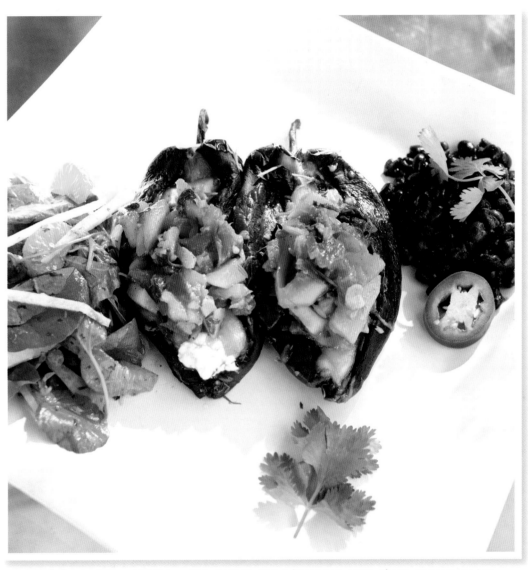

^ CILANTRO AWARD-WINNING THREE-CHEESE CHILE RELLENOS WITH FRESH PAPAYA SALSA

CILANTRO AWARD-WINNING THREE-CHEESE CHILE RELLENOS WITH FRESH PAPAYA SALSA

Chiles are known to contain capsaicin, which releases endorphins into the brain to help cure depression and anxiety. Also, there's more vitamin C found in a chile than in an orange.

Ever since I was little, I've adored my dad's chile relleno recipe. The recipe looks long, but is actually quick, easy and delicious. Perfect for a healthy Mexican fiesta!

SERVES 6

4 tsp/20 ml extra virgin olive oil

3 tbsp/20 g curry powder

¼ cup/60 g fresh ginger root, chopped

1 large red tomato, diced

6 organic poblano chiles

½ bunch of cilantro

1 firm papaya, chopped into squares

1 mango, diced

1 cup/120 g goat cheese, chopped

1 cup/120 g light Mozzarella cheese, shredded

1 cup/120 g sharp cheddar cheese, shredded

1 cup/160 g black beans, cooked

Sour cream or crème fraiche

(continued)

+ Preheat the broiler/oven on high. Pour olive oil into sauté pan and set flame temperature to medium. Add curry powder and chopped ginger to pan and sauté until ginger shows signs of browning. Depending on your stove, this could take between 5 and 10 minutes. Add diced tomato to pan, whisking to combine with curry and ginger.

While the salsa is cooking, rub chiles with some extra virgin olive oil and place on sheet pan. Place pan in the oven to blister the chiles. While the chiles are blistering in the oven, return to the salsa.

Whisk cilantro, papaya and mango together with ingredients in sauté pan. Reduce heat to a simmer until cilantro, papaya and mango are showing signs of being cooked through. This should take about 5 to 10 minutes. Remove the salsa from the heat.

Turn the chiles once while they're blistering. The sound of the chiles popping is a good sign; it means the skin is separating from the chile. Remove the chiles after about 5 to 6 minutes and place them in a brown paper bag folding over the top of the bag to steam them. After 5 to 10 minutes, remove the chiles from the bag and, under slow-running, lukewarm water, peel tough, outer skin away from one opened side of each chile. Carefully remove the seeds under the water. Using gloves is an option; sometimes the heat is harsh on hands.

Pat dry chiles with paper towel.

Place the three cheeses in a bowl and toss together. Stuff each chile with the cheese mixture. Return the stuffed chiles to the sheet pan and place the pan under the broiler until the three-cheese blend is completely melted, about 3 to 6 minutes. Remove the chiles from the broiler/oven.

Add approximately 4 tablespoons/40 g of papaya salsa to the top of each chile. Garnish with three sprigs of cilantro leaf. Serve with a side of black beans topped with a dollop of sour cream or crème fraiche.

LEMON LOVE SALMON

Salmon is an amazing source of protein and contains tons of vitamins and minerals. Add some quinoa and broccoli to this dish and it's a serious life changer. This is a meal that deserves to be cooked at least once a week.

If you don't finish all the salmon in one sitting, save it for the next day and throw it on a salad.

SERVES 2

2 salmon fillets, grilled

1 tsp/5 ml palm oil

Sea salt, to taste

Black pepper, to taste

Cayenne powder, to taste

Chili flakes (optional)

1 cup/80 g quinoa, cooked according to package directions

½ head of broccoli, chopped and steamed

1 lemon

20 capers

6 stems of rosemary

+ Preheat oven to 450°F/230°C. Rub the salmon fillets with a dime-size amount of palm oil. Season with salt, pepper and cayenne powder. Optional: Add chili flakes for a spicier dish. Place the salmon on a broiling sheet and bake in preheated oven for 5 minutes.

Change the heat temp to 500°F/260°C and turn salmon. Broil for another 5 minutes.

Arrange a bed of cooked quinoa and broccoli on a plate. Place salmon fillet on top. Squeeze lemon juice on top of the fillet and garnish with lemon slices. Add capers on top with a little extra dash of cayenne powder. Garnish with a few sprigs of rosemary.

THE RADDEST "FAKE PASTA" ON THE PLANET

My stepmom first introduced me to pasta replacements. I replace actual pasta all the time. She totally got me hooked on spaghetti squash and fresh marinara sauce. Every once in a while, she uses homemade pesto sauce, and it's like I died and went to heaven.

Anyway, lately, instead of using spaghetti squash, I've been obsessed with grilled bell peppers.

Yes, that's right. Grilled bell peppers instead of noodles. This is a great recipe for the kiddos. Most of them won't even know the difference.

NOTE: Use a slicer for best results.

SERVES 2

1 red bell pepper, sliced

1 yellow bell pepper, sliced

1 green bell pepper, sliced

1 orange bell pepper, sliced

2 tbsp/30 ml palm oil

2 handfuls broccolini, chopped

Fresh, all-natural marinara sauce

½ jalapeño, diced

½ lemon, squeezed

A sprinkle of chili flakes (if you like extra spice, like me)

Fresh basil, chopped

Optional: a few sprinkles of grated Parmesan cheese (no need for 10 handfuls)

+ Grill sliced bell peppers with palm oil in a sauté pan. Add broccolini to the pan, then the marinara sauce. Throw in jalapeños last (I like them crunchy). Transfer to a bowl. Add lemon juice, throw in chili flakes and add fresh basil. Garnish with fresh Parm. Feel free to add more sliced bell peppers!

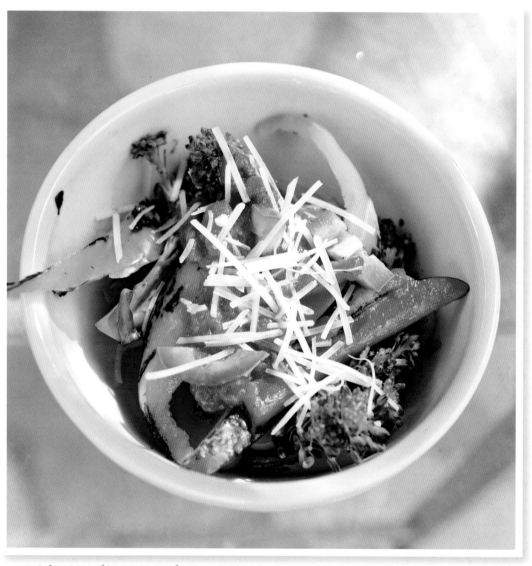

∧ THE RADDEST "FAKE PASTA" ON THE PLANET

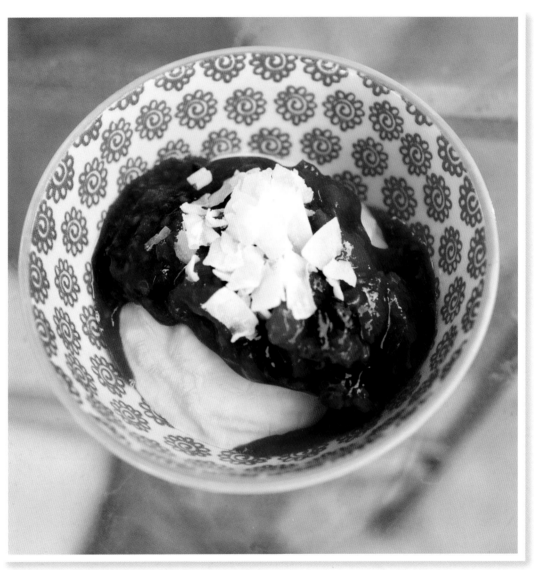

∧ BERRIES OVER ICE

>DESSERTS

BERRIES OVER ICE

I need dessert. Something sweet to end the night is essential. One of my go-to treats requires only four ingredients. This dessert is perfect for a nightcap while watching trashy TV. Enjoy!

SERVES 1

A handful of any kind of berries
1 tbsp/20 g raw honey
1 scoop of coconut yogurt
3 tbsp/14 g unsweetened coconut flakes

+ Squish berries with a fork until they appear sauce-like. Drizzle the berry sauce and honey over a scoop of coconut yogurt. Sprinkle unsweetened coconut flakes on top. If you want it sweeter, add a natural sweetener such as Stevia or a bit of raw honey.

PEANUT BUTTER "ICE CREAM"

I'm not into ice cream with 10 million ingredients. I prefer to keep it simple/stupid and know exactly what I'm putting into my bod. This guilt-free "ice cream" is seriously amaze—and for the kiddos, too!

SERVES 1

1 banana
½ **cup/90 g of peanut butter (100% pure peanut butter with no added crap)**

+ Mix banana and peanut butter together using a blender. Add mixture to a bowl. Put the skinny ice cream in the freezer for about two hours.

>SNACKS

THE ASS TIGHTENER

Let's be honest: It's difficult to find time to eat healthy. One of the best tips ever is making a smoothie the night before. Genius, right? Just freeze this recipe the night before. Make sure you leave space in the top of the glass, though, and use a freezer-safe cup. In the A.M., take it out of the freezer and enjoy as a midday snack.

SERVES 1

1 handful of baby kale

1 handful of blueberries

⅓ banana

Juice of ½ grapefruit

¼ cup/60 ml water

1 handful of ice

Optional: Grapefruit slice. For a spicy smoothie, add diced jalapeños.

+ Blend together, adding more water if needed. Garnish with a grapefruit slice.

>SKINNY COCKTAILS
BLOOD ORANGE SKINNY MARGIE-POOS

I can speak confidently on cocktails because I've been a bartender, so playing around with favors is nothing new.

My motto on margaritas is this: Use only fresh ingreds—no chemicals. No artificial shit. Absolutely none.

Stay away from store-bought margarita mix and stick with fruit.

After you have a margarita with real ingredients, you'll never go back to fake, chemical crap.

SERVES 2

2 ½ oz/70 ml 100% agave tequila

4 organic limes

2 lemons

Juice of 1 blood orange (If they're out of season, use 2 tangerines or 1 grapefruit.)

½ packet of Stevia or 1 tbsp/20 g raw organic honey

2 handfuls of ice

2 sprigs of rosemary, for garnish

Optional: Rim your glass only ⅓ of the way with salt, because is it really necessary to rim the entire glass? No.

+ Pour all the ingreds over ice in a cocktail shaker. Shake, shake, shake. Rim your glass with a lime and put salt on ⅓ of the rim. Add ice to a cocktail glass. Pour the margarita contents over the ice in the glass. Garnish with two sprigs of rosemary.

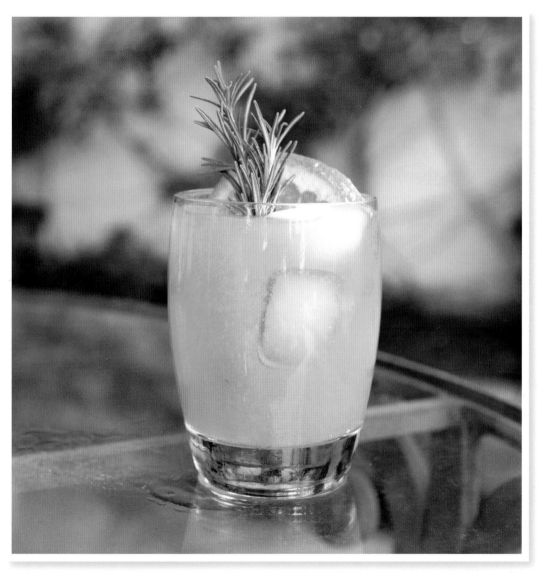

^ BLOOD ORANGE SKINNY MARGIE-POOS

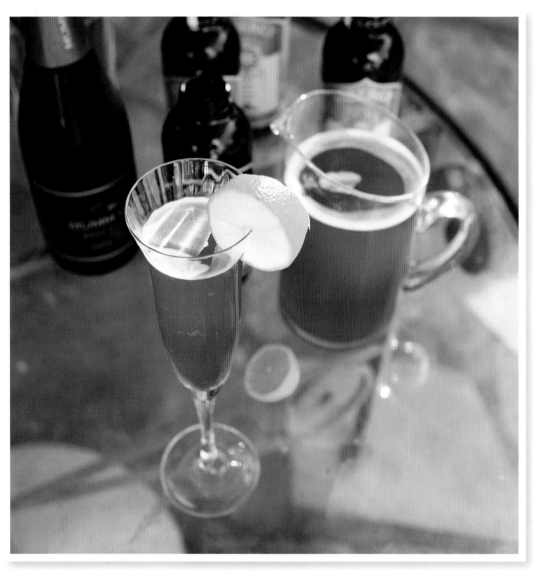

^ GETTIN' FIZZY WITH IT: A KOMBUCHA SPRITZER

GETTIN' FIZZY WITH IT: A KOMBUCHA SPRITZER

Oh hey, probiotics!

Kombucha is so cool.

Many people call it an "immortal health elixir."

Let me give you the background on this weird, delicious drink. It's refreshing and loaded with benefits. It's fermented by a bacteria and yeast culture (that's what those floaty things are at the bottom). The tea is known to help with digestion, aid with liver function, stimulate the immune system and speed the metabolism. Look for the brands with no added sugar, though (think raw kombucha—no pasteurization, please!).

So why not add a little booze to your kombucha? Check it:

SERVES 1

6 oz/170 ml dry champagne
⅓ cup/80 ml kombucha (<<< filled with probiotics!)
ice
1 lemon

+ Use a wine glass. Pour champs and your favorite flavor kombucha (I'm a fan of the guava) over ice. Add 2 squeezes of lemon and garnish with a lemon wheel. If you want to get all cute and pretty, add a colorful, striped straw!

THE POM POM LUSH

If you're a vodka-tonic lover, then get ready to shed a tear, because this info will make you never want to drink tonic again (sorry).

Tonic is filled with sugar. Yes, sugar. And sugar makes you want more sugar. You're setting yourself up with tonic. It's not just some clear, harmless liquid. It's not like soda water.

Again, sorry to be the bearer of bad news.

There's more.

Studies suggest that tonic is very similar to soda (don't even get me started on soda; I'd rather drink tar). These studies have also suggested that drinks like soda can cause weight gain and type 2 diabetes.

If you're heaving a big sigh of relief right now because you drink diet tonic, hold up.

You're definitely not in the safe zone.

Diet tonic water is sick.

It's known to increase the risk of strokes, plus it's filled with artificial sweeteners (that's what we call not eating clean).

If you're going to drink alcohol, at least make sure you're adding the freshest ingreds possible. Don't add more artificial crap to something that's already not beneficial to your health (booze).

OK, back to the recipe. This one's for the vodka lovers. I've never been big on the vod.

I mean, essentially it tastes like nothing.

I'd rather have a little bite (hi, tequila!).

This one's a quick, easy cocktail recipe that actually contains antioxidants: pomegranate seeds (not the concentrated juice, the seeds).

ice
½ lime, squeezed
1 ½ oz/40 ml vodka (my preference: Chopin)
3 oz/80 ml sparkling water
½ handful of pomegranate seeds, mashed

+ Fill a cocktail glass with ice and squeeze organic lime over the ice. Add vodka and pour sparkling water over the vodka. Mash the pomegranate seeds with a fork for about 30 seconds. You want the pom seeds to appear jam-like. Pour the mashed seeds into your cocktail. Garnish with a slice of lime. Cheers!

EXTRA ALC TIPS

Wine: Add ice to your white wine to drink it more slowly. The ice melts, leaving water in the glass, which I've found takes me longer to drink! It will also give you that extra kick of hydration.

Beer: Go for light beer. Avoid heavy, darker beers. Two of my favorites are Amstel Light® and Corona Light®. And, obviously, always add a lime so you can at least feel like you're getting some health benefits (antioxidants!!).

>SAUCES

NAUGHTY STEAK MARINADE

1.5 oz/40 ml rye whiskey
3 oz/80 ml balsamic vinegar
3 dashes of chili flakes, to taste
Sea salt, to taste

+ Mix together. Marinade time: 40 to 60 minutes.

My all-time fav salad dressing is the one on page 36. It's low cal, delish and easy to make. And a big FYI: Homemade dressings can take, like, 5 seconds to make. There's absolutely no reason to buy "low-cal" dressings filled with additives and chemicals. Homemade is the way to go! Even at restaurants, I ask for a side of lemon and chili flakes and have the waiter dress my salad in olive oil and red wine vinegar. Squeeze the lemon and chili flakes on top of the dressed salad.

There's absolutely no reason to douse your foods in caloric sauces, dressing and/or condiments. Die-hard ketchup lovers, I'm talking to you!. If you're having only a small amount, that's fine. But if you're squirting ketchup down your throat, it's probably time to find a ketchup substitution.

I mean, if your lettuce is constantly swimming in dressing, you have more cream than coffee in your cup and your French fries are becoming the condiment to your ketchup, then start to introduce your palate to the amazing world of seasoning.

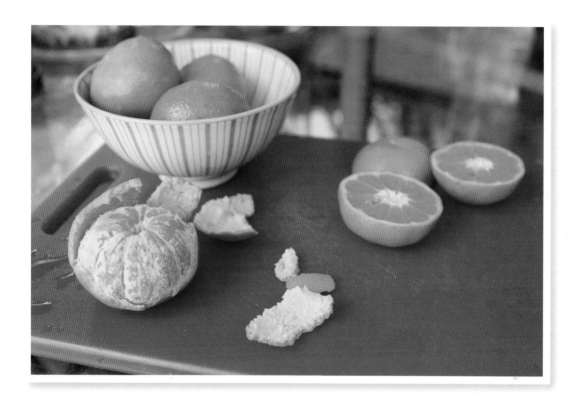

SPICES, CITRUSES AND HERBS! OH MY!

SPICE IT UP!

Cinnamon: regulates blood sugar, helps with Aunt Flow pains and reduces pain linked to arthritis.

Chili flakes: the ultimate metabolism speeder.

SEXY CITRUSES

Lemon: aids with digestion, cleanses the system and is one of the best sources for potassium.

Lime: known to reverse signs of aging, contains calcium and helps lower cholesterol.

Orange: one of the healthiest foods in the world. Oranges are a fab source of vit C and they're an amaze source of fiber.

MY FAVORITE FRESH HERBS

Basil: known to prevent some cancers and boost the immune system.

Cilantro: the best anti-inflammatory. Ever. 'Nuff said.

Rosemary: one of the best mood elevators, it freshens the breath and promotes hair growth. Sold!

Thyme: known to help relieve coughs/sore throats/colds. It's been used as a mouthwash and topical application for centuries, too.

People don't understand the power of spices, citruses and herbs. I stay away from heavy steak sauces; thick, store-bought dressings; and overly sugary condiments.

And honestly? It's not because I'm depriving myself.

It's because I'm addicted to all-natural seasonings.

Once you start to eat clean, your body (and mind) will crave clean eating automatically. It becomes a lifestyle.

For instance:

Use cinnamon, nutmeg and pumpkin pie spice in your coffee rather than artificial sweetener or sugar. Yes, there's such thing as pumpkin pie spice. It contains cinnamon, nutmeg, ginger and allspice.

Instead of mounds of ketchup, eat pico de gallo, fresh salsa or salsa verde.

Instead of tomato paste in spaghetti, make your own DIY sauce. Simply chop up fresh tomatoes with garlic, fresh basil, lemon juice, sea salt and chili flakes.

VOILÀ! SO EASY.

Know what the hell you're putting into your mouth!

Simply eat clean. Stay away from chemicals. Fuel your body with healthy, organic, fresh foods. Definitely treat yourself. But practice portion control. I say it over and over again because it's important.

Moderation is key, babes. Key.

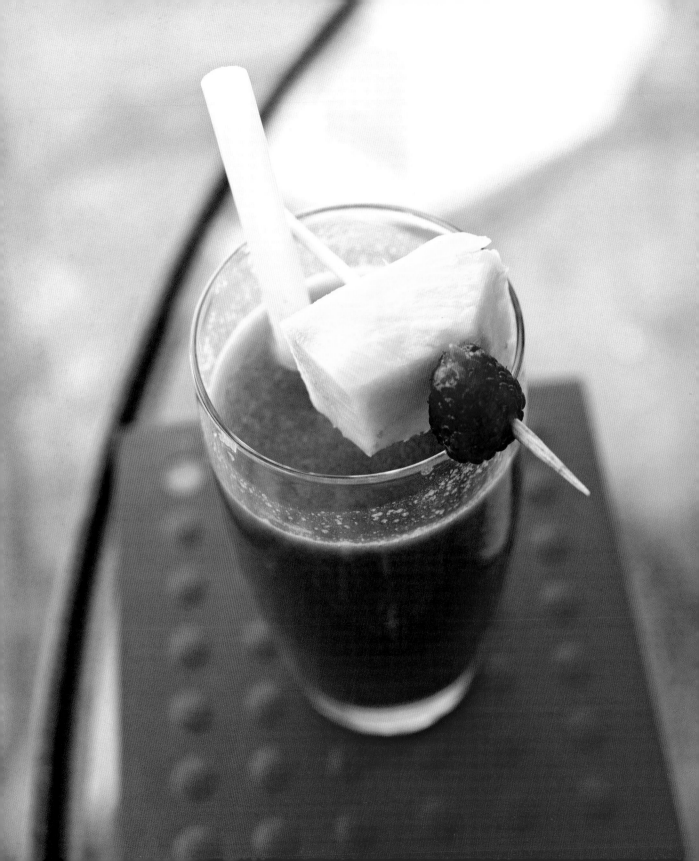

4

GREEN
POTION

Everyone should have a forever-lasting love affair with green juice.

It really is a game changer.

Ya, ya, I know what you're thinking.

TOO TRENDY!

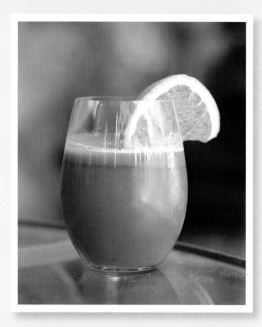

THE SKINNY CONFIDENTIAL SEXY MAGIC ELIXIR

2 handfuls of kale

½ **cucumber**

½ **grapefruit (just the juice)**

½ **lemon (just the juice)**

½ **ginger root, diced and peeled**

½ **jalapeño**

A sprinkle of cayenne on top

+ Juice everything together.

But wait.

This trend is here to stay.

Why? It will change your skin, hair, nails, diet and health.

Investing in a juicer is investing in your future.

After a while of using generic veggies, you'll start to have fun with it.

Some fun additions: turmeric, cayenne, jalapeños, ginger root, ginseng, chia seeds, hemp seeds, bee pollen, papaya...I could go on for hours.

My morning elixir kicks my ass into gear every.single. day. I never miss my daily green drink.

It's so easy after you get the hang of it. Have your ingreds prepared the night before and ready to juice in the A.M. No excuses!

If you're in a rush and can't get fresh juice, make sure you're purchasing pre-made juice that's cold pressed.

None of that pasteurized shit. 'K?

Because if juice is pasteurized, it's pretty much empty cals. And totally not clean eating (or juicing). If you're buying juice from the store, make sure it's cold-pressed and organic.

And don't even get me started on concentrated juice.

I mean, concentrated juice is just nasty. It's pumped with fillers, fake as a tanning-bed tan and filled with high fructose corn syrup. Drinking this much sug on a regular basis can cause all kinds of crazy diseases (kidney disease and diabetes to name just a couple).

RIGHT?

I can't really think of anyone who's a fan of filler in their morning OJ.

I'm so addicted to juicing, I pour a little juice over my Chihuahua's all-natural kibble every morning. Obsessed much?

Oh? You're not addicted yet?!

Hey, just because it's a dark-green icky color that you're not used to doesn't mean it tastes nasty.

First of all, man the F up!

Beauty is pain. People try new things every day to stay young and look beautiful.
Why not be beautiful from the inside out? Take care of your entire system and let it shine from the inside to the outside.

The benefits will be way worth it.

Besides, if you're so grossed out, plug your nose and drink it down the hatch. Drinking your greens is def an acquired taste, but lemme tell ya, it's one that you'll learn to love. After a while, you'll become addicted to green juice. Don't believe me? Try it!

OK, let's talk about juice cleanses.

CLEANSES ARE AMAZING.

I mean, they require some major discipline. But doesn't anything that's worth it require discipline?

You have to really get into a mindset. But any cleanse I'm a part of includes food. I like cleanses that incorporate sweet potatoes, avocados, veggies and lots of kale!

Personally, I'm a big fan of the three-day juice cleanse. I think it's just enough. Not too short, not too long.

Drinking juice all day long is so hydrating that by day three, you'll be buzzing off the walls. Cleansing flushes all the toxins out of the system. So ya, you'll probably clean out your pipes.

But who doesn't need to clean out the pipes every so often?

If you complete a cleanse properly, your stomach will shrink, your skin will shine and you'll crave healthier foods.

Make sure if you're cleansing that you're drinking tons of water, avoiding strenuous workouts (aim for Pilates and/or a light hike or walk) and getting enough sleep.

DIY Cleanse Ingredients (using 3 to 4 of each ingredient):
Day 1: cucumber, kale, apple, lemon and ginger
Day 2: beets, lettuce, carrots, celery, lemon and parsley
Day 3: apples, celery, spinach, cucumber, lemon and ginger
(Cleanse details courtesy of Juicers in Solana Beach, California)

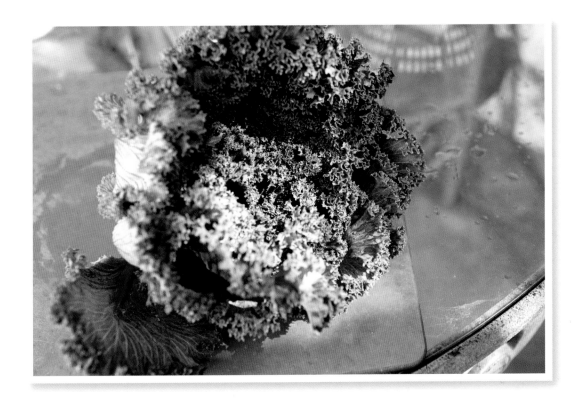

FREQUENTLY ASKED QUESTIONS ABOUT CLEANSING

I am making my juice at home; can I use a blender?

Any large juicer or blender will work. Just make sure it's large—there's a lot to hold. I use the Bella 13695 NutriPro™ Cold Press Juicer. You don't need to drink the pulp if you're using a juicer.

How much and how often do I drink the juice?

The cleanse calls for 64 ounces/2 liters a day. You drink 8 ounces/240 milliliters every hour, for 8 hours, with a cup (8 oz/240 ml) of water in between each hour. You can make the 64 ounces/2 liters the night before or the morning of. Keep in mind, the longer the juice is exposed to the air the more nutrients it loses.

Let's talk working out.

I would have a glass of orange juice (<< real, fresh orange juice, like the 100 percent, no added-shit orange juice) in the morning, especially if you're planning to work out while doing it. The only workout that I would stay away from is hot yoga. The temperature of hot yoga can be dangerous while cleansing.

I try to work out for an hour all three days of the cleanse. Think Pilates, spinning, hiking, barre classes, etc..

Explain the recipe!

This is a three-day juice cleanse. It's three to four veggies of each, depending on size. For lemons, use 3 lemons, juiced. Your veggies may be smaller than those in California, so if it doesn't make 64 ounces/2 liters, add more veggies. The skins can be peeled on certain veggies, especially carrots, beets and ginger root. All produce should be raw. Nothing should be cooked.

NOTE: Apples should NOT be blended or juiced with their seeds; they contain cyano compounds, which are carcinogenic in high enough amounts.

All veggies and fruits should be raw/uncooked.

For things like parsley and lettuce, use about three heaping handfuls. Celery is three full sticks. No canned veggies; try to use all fresh produce. I like to start drinking the juice around 9 a.m.

I always add tons of ice each time I drink the juice. It tastes SO much better that way.

I recommend doing the cleanse for only three days. If you want to detox longer, talk to your doc.

I am too busy to make the juices at home; any other options?

Yes. If you have a Whole Foods nearby, go to its juice bar or any juicing place around you. I recommend choosing that route over making it at home, it's annoying to deal with all the ingredients.

I have a number of friends who took the instructions to a Whole Foods or juice bar and it worked out well. If the juice bar doesn't have the particular veggies you're looking for, buy them yourself and take them to the counter.

If you're making the juice at home, store it in an empty, clean milk gallon. You can make it the night before if you need to. Some of my friends have also stored their juice in water bottles to drink on the go. I do not recommend juicing as you drink it. The best thing to do is wake up and make the juice each morning of days one, two and three.

So what about protein and veggies during the cleanse?

You're allowed 6 ounces/170 g of protein a day with a heaping, large handful of veggies. Here's the fab thing about this cleanse: You can have your protein and veggies **whenever you want**. For instance, one poached egg in the morning, some avocado and then ½ sweet potato at night. Stay away from red meat, if possible. My cleanse choices: lots of avocado (w/lemon and cayenne pepper) and steamed sweet potato slices throughout the day, too. Hard-boiled eggs are great for protein on the go. Not so bad, eh?

Stay away from dairy, nuts, carbs, red meat and artificial sugars.

What liquids can I drink?

No coffee, no alcohol, no sugary drinks, no soda. You should be consuming at least 3 quarts/3 L of water a day on the cleanse.

Green tea is fab. One of my tricks is a Trenta (31 oz/1 L, the biggest size available at Starbucks) of iced green tea with two splashes of passion fruit tea, no sweeteners and light on the water. I drink one or two of these a day on the cleanse.

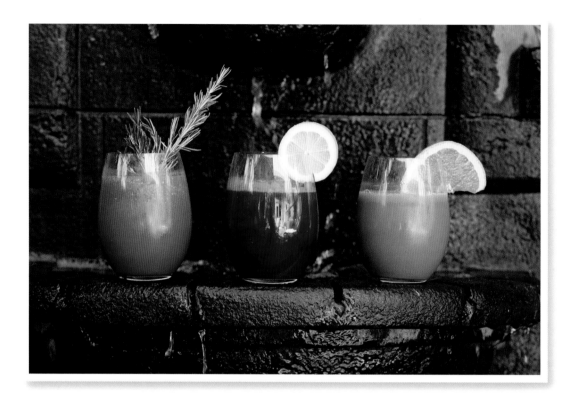

It tastes bad to me. What the hell should I do?

If you cannot stand the taste of a juice on a particular day (each day is a different flavor of juice), squeeze a ton of lemon into it to neutralize the taste. Sometimes I'll add extra ginger root, too.

I am starving on the cleanse.

If you're dying—which you shouldn't be—have an egg, a salad with red vinegar or a glass of OJ with half-sparkling water. Eating avocado slices and sweet potato slices always works, too! Make sure you're drinking the cleanse juice every hour (with tons of WATER).

How often can I do a cleanse and can I take vitamins while cleansing?

I like to do it four or five times a year. Doing it too much will not shock your body as much. You don't really need vitamins while detoxing. Your body is getting enough nutrients.

Cleansing isn't for everyone: If you have any medical conditions before, during or after the cleanse, **please consult a doctor immediately.**

One of the best ways to get all the important vitamins, minerals, enzymes, phytochemicals and amino acids you need to look and feel your best is drinking organic, raw, cold-pressed fruit and vegetable juices. That sounds pretty complicated, but it's actually pretty simple. Juices prepared this way are as clean and pure as it gets. Suja, a San Diego-based juice company, makes it extremely simple and delicious. They start with the highest-quality fresh ingredients sourced from organic and non-GMO verified farms. After washing, the produce is cold-pressed. Cold presses are different from other types of juicers because they extract juice by grinding and pressing fruits and vegetables without adding heat. In other traditional models, the fast-spinning blades that tear apart produce create heat and draw air in, allowing the juice to oxidize and killing nutrients before it even hits your cup. Sounds great, right? It is, but unless you drink your cold-pressed juice within a few hours, all those vital nutrients you worked hard to preserve are oxidizing and being minimized by heat and light. Suja takes it a step further by preserving all of the cold-pressed good-ness without applying heat as with flash pasteurization, which is used on most commercial juices. Instead of pasteurizing, Suja cold pressurizes, or HPPs, their juices. This technology, which applies a large amount of pressure to the bottles while they are kept under 40°/4°C, allows the juice to retain all of its important nutrition while extending the shelf life for 30 days and making it safe to drink as a raw product. Pretty cool.

I have friends who have cured their psoriasis, allergies and viruses by drinking the proper juices.

So do your research. Know what the hell you're chugging. Because honestly? It could just change your life.

(See Chapter 11, "Love Chub," for more of my favorite green drinks.)

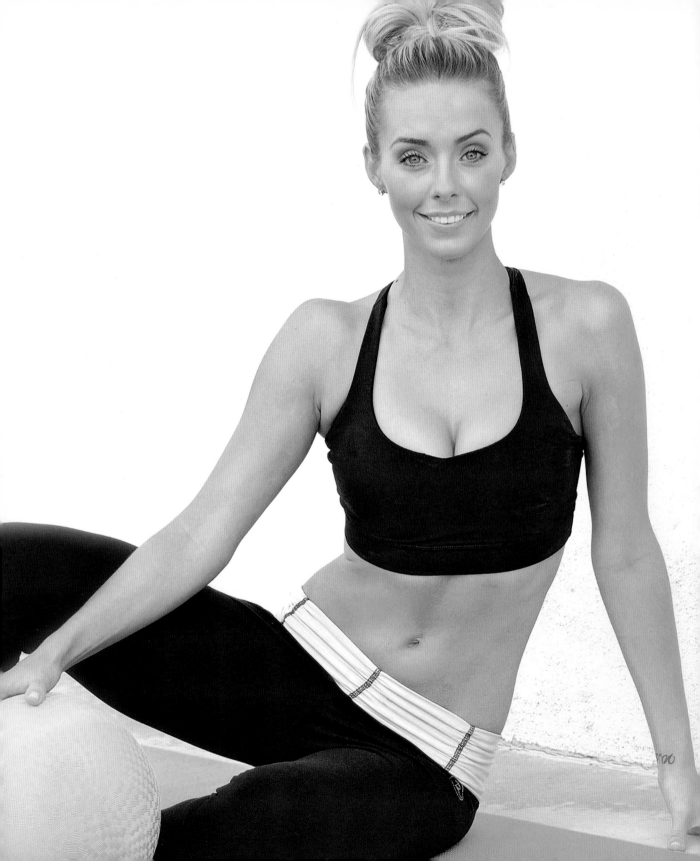

5

MEET CARDIO,
YOUR NEW BESTIE

Ahhhh, cardio.

You're such a little bitch.

My body craves you. But you're so damn difficult.

BUT, SERIOUSLY.

You're boring and repetitive.

I have to say, though, when I hang out with you, cardio, I'm tighter, leaner and longer.

Ugh. Annoying.

For now, I'll keep you around. Only three times a week, though.

'K?

xo. Lauryn

So, ya.

And that pretty much sums up my relationship with boring old cardio.

If you love cardio, you're one lucky kitten.

I've taken month breaks from boring cardio and incorporated only weight, Pilates and yoga into my daily exercises.

And let me just say: There's absolutely, positively, freaking nothing like cardio.

Cardio's a huge part of the healthy lifestyle puzzle.

Frequent cardio sesh's allow all that hard work to shine. All those toning sessions/reformer Pilates and barre classes/yoga moves will shine brighter, hunny, because you'll be tighter.

I'm telling ya, it's a real fat burner.

Plus, it releases an amazing amount of endorphins, which are vital to healthy living.

There's really no feeling like the post-cardio feeling.

LIKE, IT'S BETTER THAN SEX.

Kind of.

But I guess sex is considered cardio . . . so . . .

OK, we're getting off topic.

Anyway, here are my three favorite ways to complete my three days per week of cardio:

RUN YOUR LIL HEART OUT.

This is obvious. We all know running's cardio. But I'd be doing you an injustice if I didn't mention running. Never in my life do I feel better than when I'm running three days a week.

Sorry.

I know a lot of people don't want to hear the cold, hard facts.

It really is that simple. So simple, it's almost stupid.

An amazing benefit of running: It's a serious metabolism speeder.

I'm into intervals. After talking to multiple fitness trainers, it seems that intervals are the way to go when it comes to running.

Why?

GLAD YOU ASKED.

Instead of running 30 minutes consecutively at a pace of 6.5 or 7.5 minutes per mile, allow your bod to recover every minute. For example: Run 1 minute at 3.5 pace and 1 minute at 6.5, increasing slowly up to 7.5 as you go. I like to run for 30 minutes total.

Allowing the body to recover through interval training will help with stress in general. Interval training allows the body to deal with stress constructively because it's taking the heart rate up and then down, and then up and then down, etc. It puts the body under stress and then allows it to recover. These stress tactics can be applied to life in general.

TAKE A HIKE

A great activity to do with friends. An even greater activity if you can cut the gossip in half and kick the speed up ten notches. Make sure you're not just using hiking as "fake cardio."

YOU KNOW, YOU KNOW.

Get your heart rate up. I'm sure you're dying to hear whose boyfriend is a scumbag, douche and what happened to Cindy last night, but if you decide to hike, then hike.

Besides, in-between breaths, I'm sure you'll be able to hear what happened on last night's epi of "Real Housewives."

Anyway, my trick to hiking is to bring arm weights. I purchased these bad boys at a superstore (think Walmart, for example). I like 5-pound/2-kg arm weights. They wrap around the arms so they're not in the way, and they can also be used as ankle weights.

Get creative! Walk half the time, run half the time. Do lunges up the hill. Skip. Stretch afterward. Side-step up.

ELLIPTICAL TRAINER, STAIR MACHINE AND/OR SPIN CLASSES

I pick one of these workouts and use it only once a week. I notice my lower body bulks up if I do too many machines or classes. I also get bored.

Again, do what works for you. If spinning keeps your stems slim, spin, spin and spin some more.

The elliptical can be great, too; however, nothing raises your heart rate like running.

Sorry, Ellipty.

GOOD OLD SPORTS

We all loved at least one sport when we were kids, right?

I definitely was and still am into tennis.

Anyway, revert back to your childhood. Pick a sport, any sport.

And go play it. Grab some friends (and most likely a ball of some sort) and get at it.

SWEATING WHILE YOU'RE HAVING FUN? THERE'S NOTHING BETTER.

A little FYI: The more creative you get with your cardio routine, the better. If you change it up frequently, the body will be shocked.

That's right. Shock the hell out of your body.

The last thing anyone wants is to be stuck in a plateau.

Plateaus are like being in a bad relationship for six months too long.

You're bored, uninspired, lazy and miserable.

Leave the plateau in the dust just like that sucky ex.

Mmkay?

So every week, switch up your workouts. If you hiked last Tuesday, run this Tuesday. If you did hot yoga on Friday, do yoga with weights on Sunday.

Mix it up.

SO, HOW OFTEN SHOULD YOU WORK OUT?

Welp, everyone's different.

All of us have different genetics, different diets and different shapes.

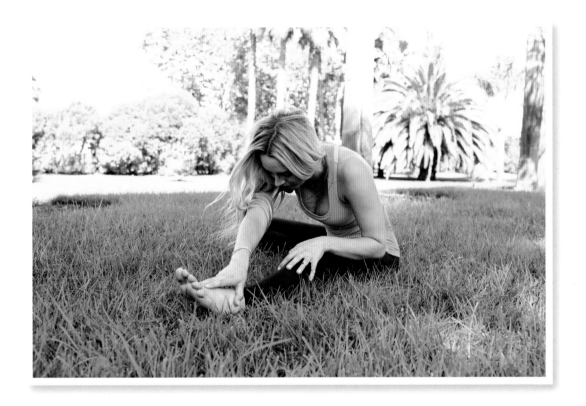

My biggest tip? Say you're going to work out seven days a week. Shooting for all seven days will force you to get in at least five or six. Plan for every day and you're bound to get more workouts in than if you planned for five workouts. Let's face it: Shit happens . . . life happens. So instead of freaking out because you have to skip yoga due to traffic, don't fret. You still have six more days of the week!

Plus, if you end up working out all seven days, you're a total star.

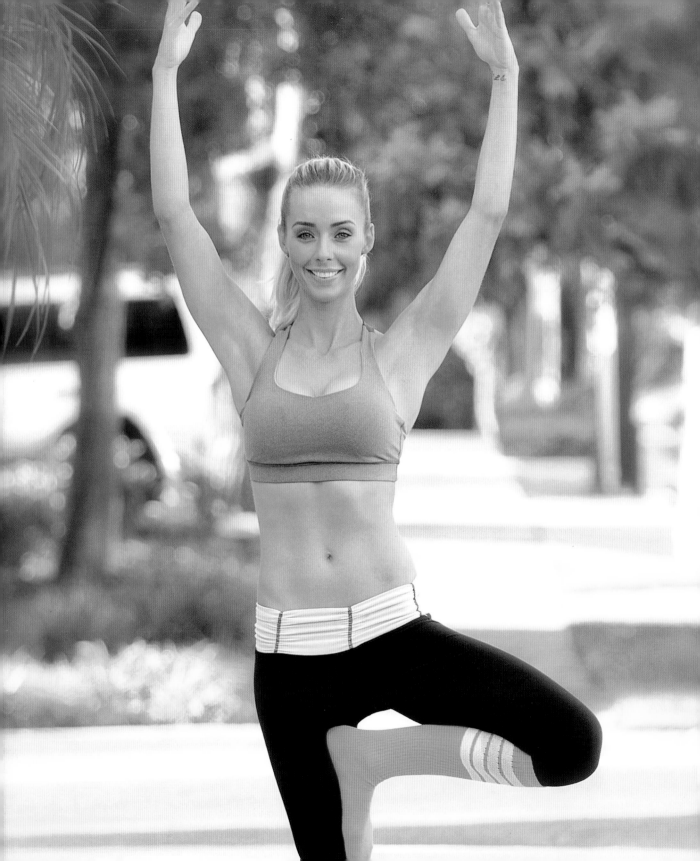

And don't forget to stretch! Yoga is obviously amazing for stretching, but I feel like many people are scared of the workout.

Scared of being in a heated room.

Scared of feeling embarrassed that they're unable to complete a full-blown "Eagle" pose.

Scared of their balls hanging in someone's face while they're in "Downward Dog." (Unless, of course, you're a woman).

Here's the deal: Find a yoga class that fits your needs. There are about a million yoga programs (beginning, advanced, heated, nonheated, stretch-related, Bikram, Ashtanga, etc.). Figure it out and try to go to a class at least once a week.

I'm not asking you to give up your firstborn; I'm just asking for an hour a week. Get your stretch on!

DOABLE?

I think so.

Plus, flexibility is an absolute necessity to living a healthy lifestyle.

It stretches the muscles to create that long, lean, lingerie model look.

Sweating and stretching go hand in hand. So pick your exercise, incorporate stretching and make sure you schedule your workouts on your calendar app.

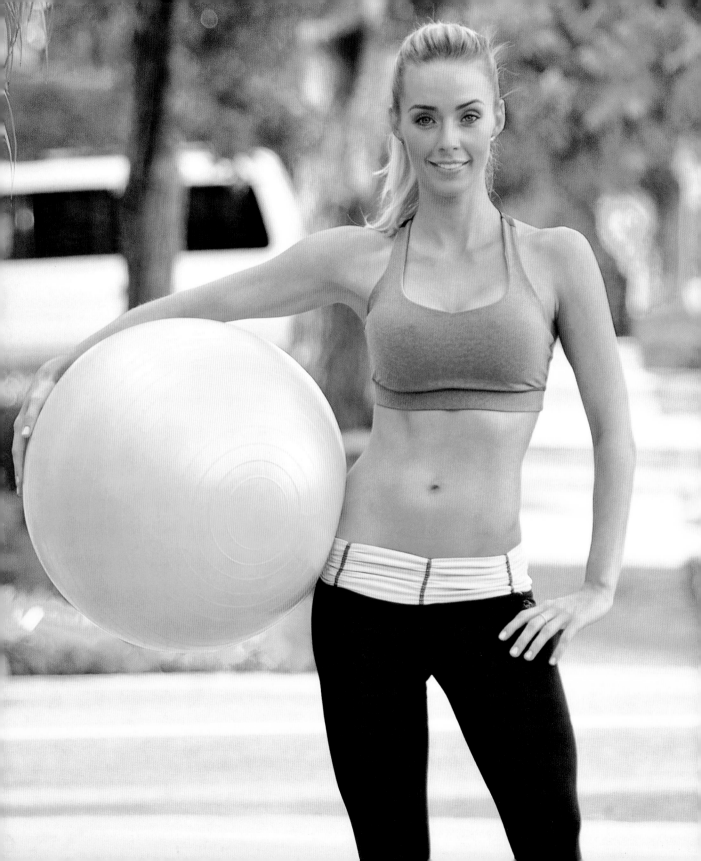

6

STRENGTH TRAINING: GET IT RIGHT, GET IT TIGHT!

First things first.

If you're one of those babes who thinks that weights equal bulk, then think again.

Sorry. It's a total myth that you should stay away from weights if you're trying to avoid bulk.

Fact: Weights can be absolutely amazing if they're used properly.

One of my favorite things about weight lifting is that it's a real metabolism booster. Light weights used correctly can take the metabolism to a different level.

MORE STRENGTH TRAINING BENEFITS:

+ Helps with concentration
+ Controls weight gain
+ Reduces signs of chronic conditions
+ Increases bone density

According to Edward R. Laskowski, M.D., a physical medicine and rehabilitation specialist at the Mayo Clinic in Rochester, Minnesota, and co-director of the Mayo Clinic Sports Medicine Center, "If you don't do anything to replace the lean muscle you lose [with age], you'll increase the percentage of fat in your body. But strength training can help you preserve and enhance your muscle mass—at any age." *(Source: www.mayoclinic.com)*

Oh! And not only am I a huge fan of big movement, but I'm also an isometric junkie.

So...WTF does isometric mean?

Isometric is when you isolate the muscle with tiny, little movements that get the tiny, little muscles that people tend to forget. So rather than completing workouts with a big range of motion, you're staying in one position for a longer period of time (in a more static position).

OK, so let's talk about specific areas of the bod.

AHEM.

We shall begin with bat wings.

If I had a dime for every time my friends called me complaining about their bat wings, I'd be richer than Richie Rich.

I mean, life doesn't always have to be so difficult. ESP when it comes to dinky, cheap 5-pound/2-kg weights.

All you have to do is grab about five dollars and head over to a store like Target or Marshall's and grab some hot little 5 pounders.

Come home, turn on some tunes, do a minimum of ten minutes a day. If you're feeling sexy and strong, try for fifteen to twenty!

EASY, RIGHT?

So, if you're interested in fixing that under-arm flab that waves in the breeze every time you say good-bye, then check out the following bat wing busters.

Because if you're buying turtlenecks over sleeveless tanks to hide your arms, it's time to take action and nip those bat wings in the bud.

NOTE: Some exercises include an upward pulse. A pulse is simply a slight push of about ½ inch/12 mm—a tiny movement while the crown of the head reaches to the sky.

BAT-WING BUSTERS:

The Bye-Bye, Arm Jiggle: Stand with your arms in an "L" position by your sides. Think of a goal post shape. Press up into an "O" shape, above your head. Make sure your shoulders are not touching your ears. Abs are pulled in tight. Use at least 5-pound/2-kg weights for this exercise. Do three sets of twenty. At the end of each set, add ten pulses upward, while still in your "O" shape.

Welcome to the Gun Show (AKA dumbbell curl): Feet are hip-width apart and parallel. Bend one arm to ninety degrees, keeping the other arm straight. As your curl, switch the arms. Do ten on each side (three sets) with at least 5-pound/2-kg weights.

Push-ups, tricep dips (off a chair) and pull-ups are also game changers when it comes to arms. My typical routine calls for 3 sets of ten slow and five fast of each exercise.

Victoria's Real Secret (AKA tricep extension): I love this particular exercise because it lengthens my abs. Pilates creates longer and leaner abs. It can also make some people grow taller by lengthening their spines, while strengthening the arms, shoulders, chest and lats. Stand with feet hip-width apart and arms straight up holding the weights. Squeeze the elbows close to the head. Lower the 5-pound/2-kg weights behind your head and then extend up toward the sky. Aim for full extension to attain those long, lean muscles. Do three sets of twenty. At the end of each set, add five pulses upward, while your arms are straight in the air.

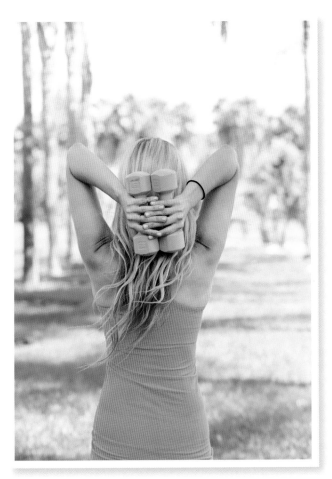

^ Stand up tall, holding the weights behind your head, elbows bent.

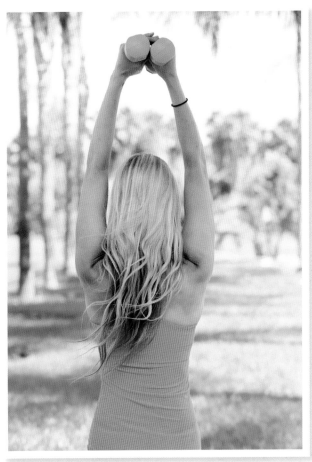

^ Extend your arms straight up.

The Flipsy-Whipsy: With 5-pound/2-kg weights in each hand, extend your arms out to the sides. You should look like a giant, lowercase "T." Flip the hands up and down. So, thumbs up, thumbs down. The slower, the better. Do three sets of fifteen. Make sure your arms are straight out from your shoulders the whole time. Take the neck out of the workout.

Perform these easy, quick arm exercises at least three times a week, and in no time your arms will be jiggle-free!

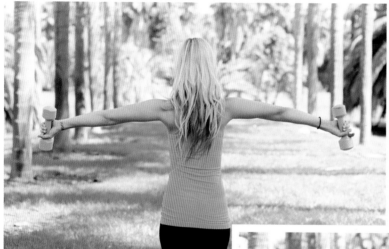

∧ Stand tall with a weight in each hand and your arms out at your sides.

∨ Flip your hands up and down.

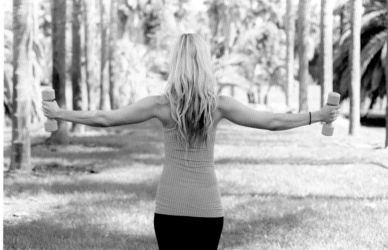

THREE EASY EXERCISES YOU CAN DO WHILE WATCHING "REAL HOUSEWIVES OF WHATEVER."

Sexy Stemmers (AKA good, old-fashioned lunges): Lunges, lunges, lunges! Tone the legs fast and efficiently by standing with your feet hip-width apart and parallel. Place your hands on your waist. Step forward with one leg and lower your body by bending both knees. Take both legs to ninety degrees. Hold for a second and switch. All the pressure should be in your heels. Do three sets of twenty at least twice a week.

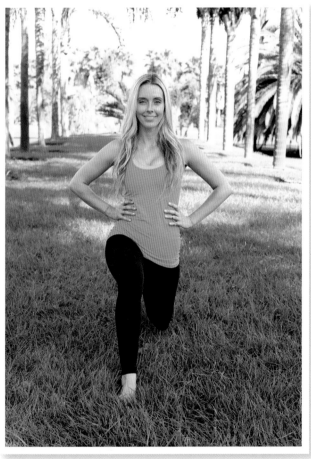

∧ Stand with your feet hip-width apart, and step forward with one leg.

Cracked-Out Squats: Feet are hip-width apart and parallel. Bend the knees, making sure to keep them in line with the butt. Hands are on the hips. After you've done twenty squats, hold the last one down and pulse gently (down and up) for thirty seconds for three sets.

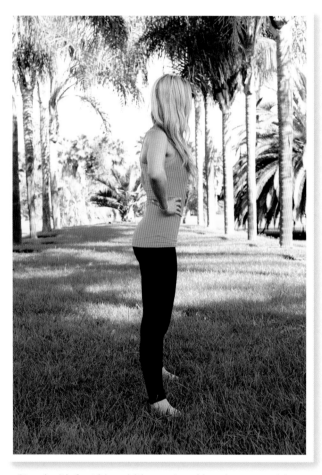

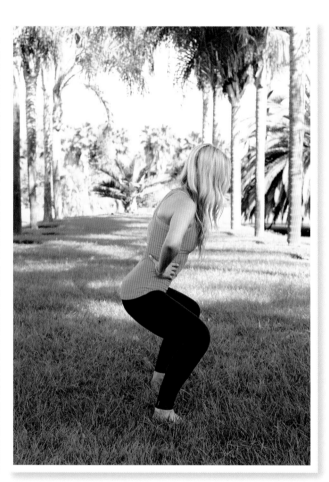

∧ Stand with feet hip-width apart and hands on your hips.

∧ Bend your knees and lower your body toward the floor.

Balls to the Walls: Grab a huge exercise ball. Press your lower back into the ball while contracting your abs. Feet are hip-width apart and parallel, hands are behind your ears. Press your spine into the ball and do a sit up. Do three sets of fifteen.

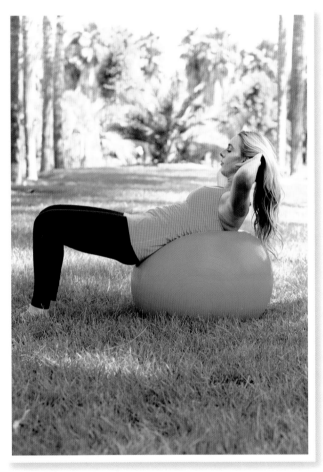

∧ Lie down on an exercise ball and do some sit ups to work your abs.

LET'S NOT FORGET ABOUT THE ASS.

If you want to tone your butt, strength training should become your overnight bestie.

Here are my favorite ways to exercise off the stuff that hangs out of the bikini:

The Butt Lifter: Come down on all fours. Kick your right leg back like a donkey and then pull it back in (leaving your left leg on the ground) for forty-five seconds. You're targeting the smile in the right side of the butt. Repeat on the left side. Do three sets.

The J.Lo: Hip lifts are key, peeps. If you're craving some curves, you'll love this one. Lie on your back with your knees bent and arms at your sides, hands pressing into the floor. Feet are hip-width apart and parallel. Press your feet into the ground as you lift your hips upward. Hold the hips up until they're aligned with your knees and spine. Hold for fifteen seconds and repeat. Do three sets of fifteen.

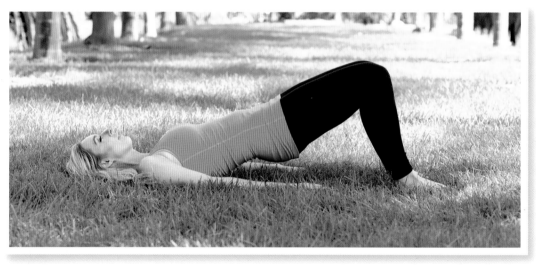

∧ **The J. Lo:** Lie on your back with your knees bent. Lift your hips upward and hold for fifteen seconds.

The Smiley Ass: Again, you're targeting the smile where the hamstring meets the butt. This is one of my favorite workouts. Come down onto all fours. Extend one leg straight to the side so it's coming diagonally off the hip. Point the toe. Take it down to the ground and then bring it slowly up to hip height. Try to even out the pressure in the forearms (or hands). Contract your seat the whole time, rolling your hips under and pulling the abdominals inward toward the spine. Do twenty on each leg (fourty total) for three sets.

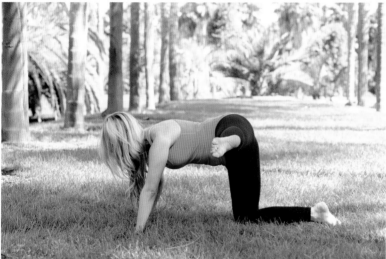

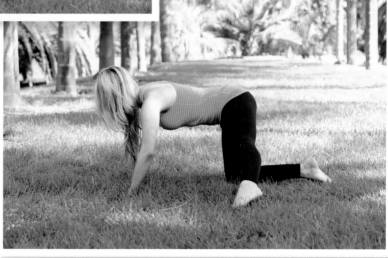

v Bring your leg to the ground and slowly lift to hip height for one rep.

∧ Come down on all fours and extend one leg straight to the side.

IF WE'RE GOING TO TALK ABOUT BUTT BUSTERS, WE NEED TO TALK ABOUT BOOBIES.

Dying to make the girls perkier? Welp, there are exercises for that, too.

YA. I WENT THERE.

Sorry, boys; this doesn't apply to you.

Fun bags are made up of fat that sits on top of the muscle, so while it's not possible to really work out your breasts, it is possible to add muscle mass to the chest area to make them appear bigger (and perkier).

HERE ARE SOME SUPER-PERKY TA-TA WORKOUTS:

Lifetime Fun Bag (AKA closed-up push ups): Get on the floor on all fours (plank position). Place your hands close together with index fingers and thumbs touching, forming a diamond on the floor. Do three sets of ten push ups in this position. If that is too hard, perform them on your knees for a modification.

A Real Hooter (using 5-pound/2-kg weights): Frame your face with the weights (one in each hand). Slowly bring your arms out to the sides, making a goal post shape. Bring your arms back in, weights touching, and that one. After completing fifteen of these, hold the weights still (out like a goal post)and pulse upward and down for forty-five seconds. Do three sets of fifteen with 45-second pulses after each.

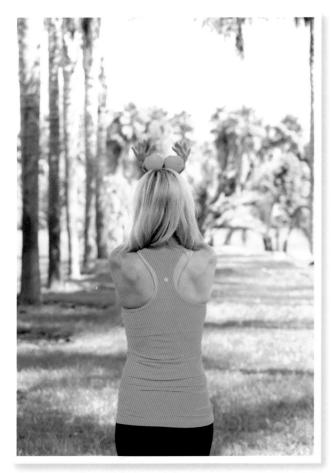

∧ Frame your face with the weights.

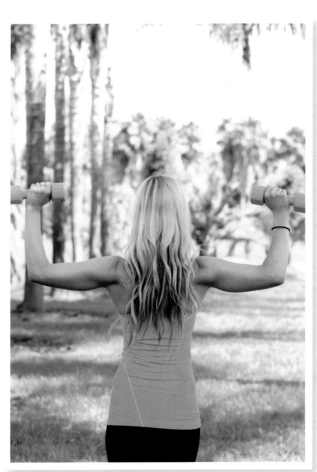

∧ Make your arms form a goal post.

The Perky McPerkinson: Grasp your weights and lie on the floor, on a bench or ball with your arms straight out from your sides, in a T position. Knuckles, wrists and arms should be in line with the shoulders. Lift the weights, bringing the knuckles together. Then bring them back to the T position, feeling a slight stretch and repeat. Complete three sets of twenty.

Later, saggiers!

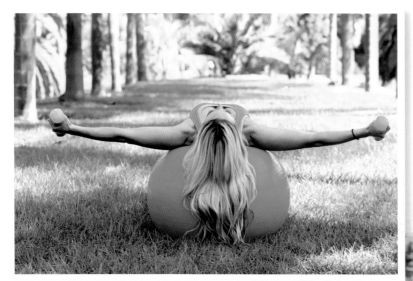

v Lift the weights, bringing your knuckles together.

^ Lie on a ball with weights in your hands, arms out from your sides.

AND LAST, BUT NOT LEAST, LET'S DISCUSS LOVE HANDLES.

Love handles are a slight bulge or puffiness that hangs out of the jeans. I mean, having small love handles is perfectly normal, but looking like your jeans are ten sizes too small because there's flab hanging off the sides is just unnecessary. Love handles can be fixed easily by diet, exercise and stress management.

A few years ago, I was not loving my love handles. So here's how I got rid of those nasty little shits:

Fiery Forearm Planks (both sides!): Easy, peasy. On the floor, in a push-up position, lower the right forearm to a 90° angle and rest your weight on it. Make sure your shoulders are out of the ears and the neck is long. You want one straight line from the crown of your head to your heels. This is a plank. Simply plank on your right forearm for one minute and then on your left forearm for one minute. Do a total of three on each forearm. This exercise tightens up the abs and obliques immediately.

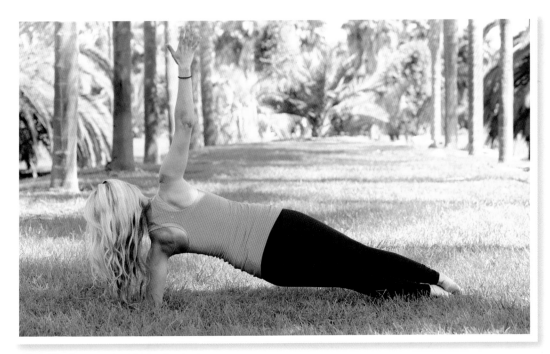

∧ Side Plank on each side for 1 minute.

The Twister: This exercise is super easy. Just sit on your tail (yes, your tailbone) with your knees bent. Legs are squeezed together tightly, and the abs are pulled in. Grab your weights and make sure your toes are off the ground and the legs are at 90 degrees. Start switching side to side. Go right to left. Do fifteen on each side, three sets. For some isometric movement, add a hold on each side for ten seconds at the end of each set.

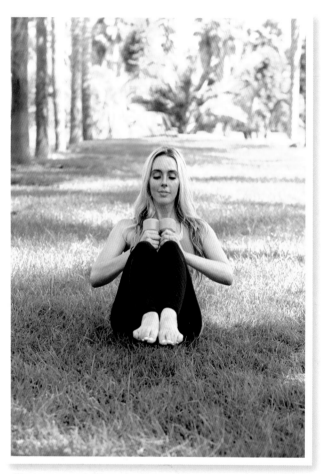

∧ Start on your tailbone with knees bent.

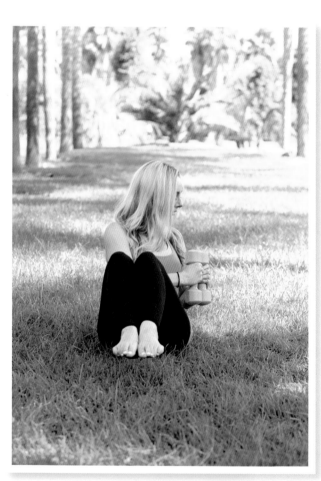

∧ Move from side to side to work your love handles.

The Love Handle Blaster: Lie down with your hands behind your head. Extend your legs stick straight. Scissor the legs, keeping the legs as straight as possible. Bring your opposite hand to the opposite foot, keeping the other hand behind your head. You can also relax the shoulders and press your hands into the ground while scissoring the legs. After completing twenty switches (ten on each side), hold the left hand to the right foot and pulse up twenty times toward the pinky toe. Then switch to the other side for twenty pulses. Do three sets.

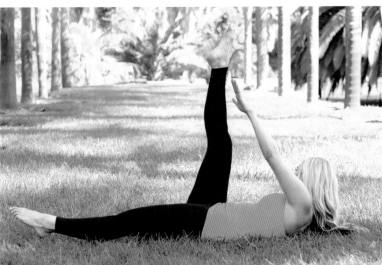

∧ Lie down flat on the floor and touch your left hand to your right foot.

∨ Then touch your right hand to your left foot.

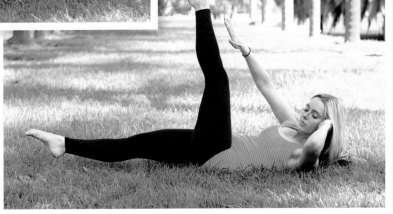

Practicing strength lifting properly really helps people learn to deal with stressful situations better. Putting your body under stress with weights for a minute and then letting your body recover for a minute from that heavy, slow resistance can also help with stress in general.

And don't forget about hormones (because honestly? Most people do!). The stress hormone cortisol is known to cause belly fat. When the body produces too much cortisol, it can increase the appetite. Pretty much, high cortisol levels = more hunger pangs. Many researchers believe that people who gain weight from stress are more likely to have belly fat.

Using weights speeds up the metabolism and helps the body recover from stressful situations. Weight lifting obviously releases endorphins into the brain. So when the happy sensation releases into the body, it relieves stress (buh-bye, cortisol!) and changes a bad mood into a happy, sexy mood.

IT'S A WIN, WIN.

I love doing strength training exercises at the beach with a couple of my girlfriends. We usually aim for two to three days a week for forty-five minutes per session. Each of us brings weights and a resistance band.

Naturally, I'm always multitasking: We gossip, sweat and enjoy the beach's fresh air.

So.

Flab, schmab. Now there's no excuse!

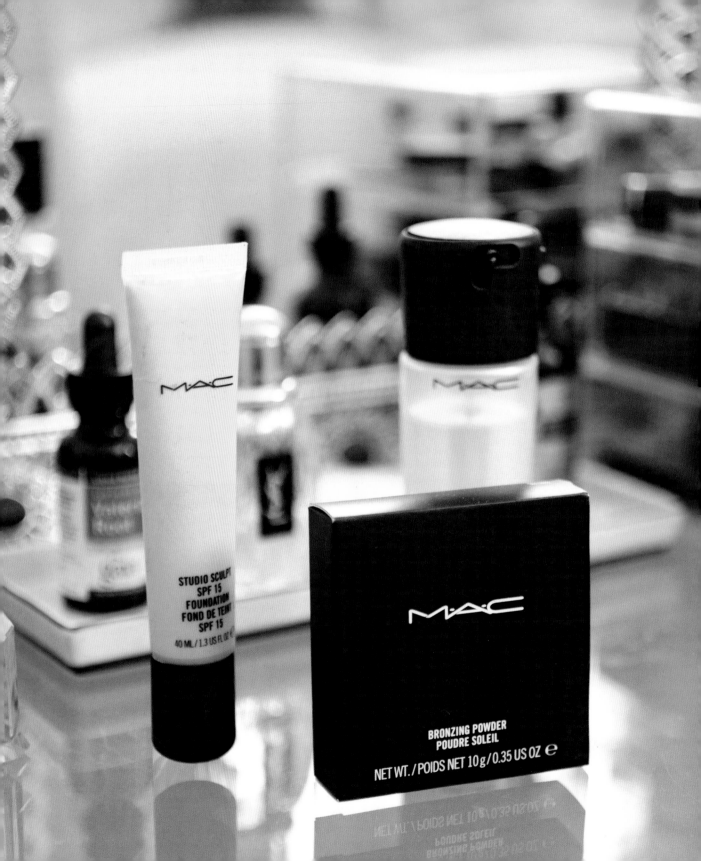

7

WTF'S IN MY

MAKEUP BAG?

Makeup is my thing. I've researched everything under the sun. But what's not my thing? Painting my face like a full-blown clown. I'm not into globs of eye shadow, dark lip liner and/or thick liquid eyeliner. Keep it fresh and simple, and let your natural beauty shine.

OK, so let's be clear: The cake face is out (I mean, was it ever in?).

Caking your face in makeup is just nasty. Guys don't like it; girls don't like it; no one likes it.

My goal with makeup is to use it to enhance my features without making me look like a completely different person.

Let's start from the beginning:

Primer: Not putting on primer before your makeup is like da Vinci not using canvas primer before painting the Mona Lisa.

Face makeup simply won't live up to its full potential without primer.

SO. USE YOUR PRIMER, BABES.

After you've cleansed your face, prepare it with a light-weight primer. Rub it all over your face. Quick, easy, simple.

Moisturizer + foundation: After your canvas is primed and ready, grab your moisturizer.

My biggest makeup tip? Mix your foundation with moisturizer.

Why?

Because it's a total game changer. Not only does it make your skin dewy, but it also takes that cakey foundation look away. To each their own, but I like to use a dime-size amount of foundation and a quarter size of moisturizer.

Buh-bye, cake face.

It's also helpful on the wallet. Mixing foundation with moisturizer will make your foundation last and last and last.

Moving on! You know what the crime of the century is? Buying foundation that doesn't have SPF.

I mean, why on earth would you choose a foundation without SPF when you can choose one with it?

BEATS ME.

When you're choosing a foundation, make sure it's a full-coverage brand with SPF. Also, please, please, please make sure it doesn't contain titanium dioxide. This disgusting, sick-o chemical's known to cause cancer.

Oh. And make sure your foundation matches your skin tone. If your body is pale, then your face shouldn't be orange. If your body is tan, your face shouldn't look like the main character in the movie "Powder." If your body is spray-tan orange, learn how to spray tan and then deal with foundation colors. The worst thing ever is when a girl has a thick line of foundation that looks similar to a mask.

Makeup 101: Rub your foundation (with your moisturizer mixed in) into your neck.

CAPISCE?

OK, now for the I-can't-live-without-it-or-I'll-die makeup tool: a foundation brush. After I've primed my face, I take my moisturizer, squeeze it on the top of my hand (about two small dapples) and then squeeze one dime-size dot of foundation on top. I mix the two together with my foundation brush. Then I pat the foundation on my face. Not only does this work for me, but it's also super fun.

I like to put more foundation on the areas that need it—i.e., under-eye circles, the middle of my forehead, the tops of my cheekbones (this makes them pop) and last, but definitely not least, my eyelids.

Painting foundation on your eyelids brightens the eyes. They'll appear cleaner and more awake. I've been doing this trick forever and I'm obsessed.

Trust me; you'll be obsessed, too.

After I've put on my moisturizer plus foundation, I let it sit.

The biggest makeup mistake girls make is not letting their foundation sit on their skin. Seriously peeps, all I'm asking for is one minute.

After it's done sitting, I use concealer. FYI: I skip the powder part. Powder makes my face look too cakey. And honestly? I'm more of a dewy girl. I like that beaming, dewy look that's fresh. Pounding powder on makes me look too done up.

OK, back to the concealer. This is a bit tricky; a lot of girls abuse poor, poor concealer. Don't give it a bad rep.

Concealer is meant to be used in small quantities and is used for covering a zit or a brown spot, not your whole face. In my opinion, a tiny bottle of concealer should last you months.

Months. Not days. Months.

I use my ring finger to pat (not rub) a few dots of concealer on any blemishes and under my eyes.

Quick tip: Use a line of concealer to frame the outside of the nose (on the cheek area, not on the actual nose) to make your nose appear smaller.

Once your concealer is applied, grab the bronzer. Pick a bronzer that isn't overly sparkly.

I MEAN, THIS ISN'T A KESHA CONCERT.

Let's keep it classy. A bit of shimmer is pretty; a boatload of glitter isn't. Save it for the slutty fairy Halloween costume.

Make sure you have a bronzer brush, not an eye shadow brush, not a foundation brush—a bronzer brush. If you decide to not use a bronzer brush, then you might as well compare it to using a curling iron to straighten your hair.

Put a bit of bronzer on the brush and apply it to your cheekbones. Where the F are your cheekbones? Try this little exercise to find them. Pretend you're drinking out of a straw and purse your lips together. You should see two prominent cheekies sticking out. Put the bronzer on them.

Then add a dot of bronzer to the underneath portion of your bottom lip. Why?

Because.

It's an amazing trick to make that lower lip appear bigger and poutier. FYI: If you're Angelina Jolie, you probably can skip this part.

If you're not Angie, then bronze on.

Add a bit more bronzer to your brush and add some bronzer to the top of your hairline, not the whole forehead.

Side note: You want to know what drives me bat shit crazy? When people put bronzer over their whole face. Not hot. Not cool. Not fun to look at.

Anyway, you can add some bronzer to the jawline, too. This will slim the chin.

Next step: Grab your highlighter. Here's the fun part: Highlight the features you love. The tops of the cheekbones are fun to highlight (above the bronzer), and a little highlighter under the brow bone is sexy. If you want that Kim K. glow, add some highlighter above your lip. You know that little dip above the top lip? That's where you want the highlighter. For a smaller nose, add it to the bone on your nose and in the middle of your forehead.

If you're into the rosy cheek look, add some cream blush to the apples of your cheeks. Keep it soft though—no need to look like a circus clown.

NOW IT'S TIME TO BLEND!

I like to use a Kabuki brush to blend. The short stem and dense bristles will blend everything together so you don't look like you used multicolored permanent markers on your face. Get excited! The Kabuki brush is God-sent. Honestly, it's a game changer.

After you've blended your face to create a masterpiece, it's time to fill in those brows. Because no one likes tadpole brows. Thick brows are in. Brows are sexy when they're full and shaped properly. If you're confused about how to shape brows, go to a waxing salon (a real waxing salon, not some weird hole in the wall). Bring pictures of what you're envisioning for your brows.

But remember: Do what works well for your face. I put my tweezers down a long time ago. I couldn't be trusted. I was a total over-plucker. If this sounds like you, step.away.from.the. tweezers. Leave it to the professionals, babes.

Back to filling in the brows. My favorite brow kit is made by Anastasia. It contains the perfect brow brush with colors that fit well with any hair color.

When it comes to filling in my brows, I make three, tiny lines: one at the beginning of the brow, one at the peak of the brow and one at the end.

Once they're filled in, I use a clear mascara to brush them. Yes, peeps. You brush your hair, you brush your teeth, you brush your brows. Common sense.

Mascara time!

Mascara is my jam. After speaking with many makeup artists, I've found that none of them know this trick:

Prime. Curl. Prime. Curl. Mascara.

Here's the deal: I would rather not put on makeup if I don't have mascara primer. I'm not talking about clear, see-through primer. I'm talking about white, thick primer (I like one from Dior). White, thick primer will make your lashes five times thicker and longer than they actually are naturally.

SO. AHEM!

My favorite makeup secret works like this:

Do one eye at a time: Prime with your white, thick primer. Curl with an amazing eyelash curler (the better the curler, the better the lash looks). Prime again. Curl again (but only if it's nighttime; once will suffice in the daytime).

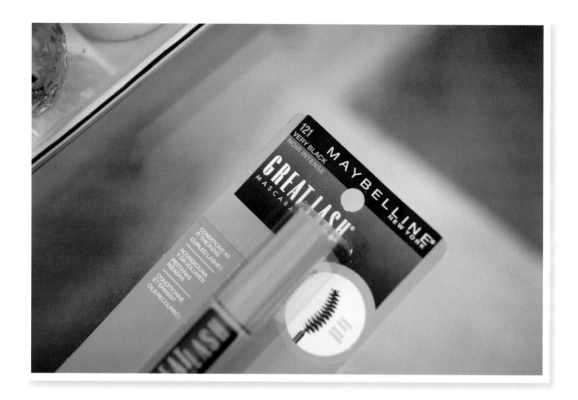

After you've primed twice and curled the lash twice, add your mascara. Listen: Mascara is funny. There are a million choices and each one promises different things (bigger lashes! longer lashes! volumized lashes!). Find one that works for you. My obsession is Great Lash® Blackest Black with a curled wand. It's four dollars at any local drugstore. I've tried every mascara under the sun. If I really want to make my lashes as long as possible, I apply Benefit's "They're Real." This particular product was sent from the mascara gods. It literally gives the illusion of fake lashes.

RAD.

After you're all mascara-ed up, grab the gloss and lip liner, sex kitten.

Add a dab of shiny gloss to the middle of your upper and lower lips. This will give you the perfect pout.

As for lip liner: I'm not talking '90s maroon lip liner from the movie "Clueless". My favorite liners are a nude and a tan. I use the nude on the top of my lips; it makes them pop. And the tan liner goes on the bottom.

The point is: It looks like I'm not wearing lip liner, but gives the illusion of a perf pout.

I mean, isn't that the whole point of makeup? To look like you're not wearing any? Keep it simple!

Anyway, there you have it. That's my makeup application process.

TA DA!

Oh! BTW: I'm not an eye shadow wearer. I don't like it. It looks gaudy on me and doesn't work for my face, but do whatever floats your boat.

This may seem like a lot of work, but the whole process should never take more than ten minutes! And, if you're going to make the effort to apply makeup every day, be sure to make the effort to take it off. The worst thing ever is waking up on a white pillow full of mixed colors.

FYI: If you're going for a sophisticated look, clear lips are amaze. A lot of gloss is very baby doll. Add some extra blush to the apples of the cheeks, too. A thick brow is also sophisticated and chic.

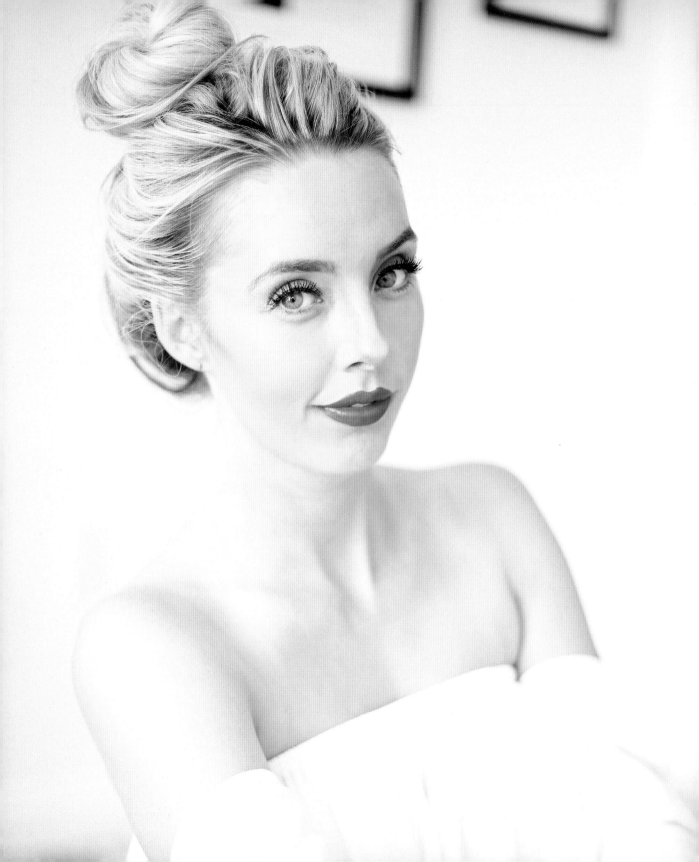

For a going-out look, I die over red, orange (yes, hot orange is fun and sassy!) and dark maroon lips. Fake eyelashes (the natural-looking ones) are always sexy to throw on for a night out on the town, too. Pull your hair back for a more dramatic look; girls who pull their hair off their faces know how to rock it. A ponytail screams confidence because you're not using your hair as a security blanket. Also, a bun or a braid is unexpected and so much more interesting than wearing your hair down.

And lastly, if you want to include some sparkle, add a headpiece!

Overall makeup lesson: The overdone look is too much—keep it natural!

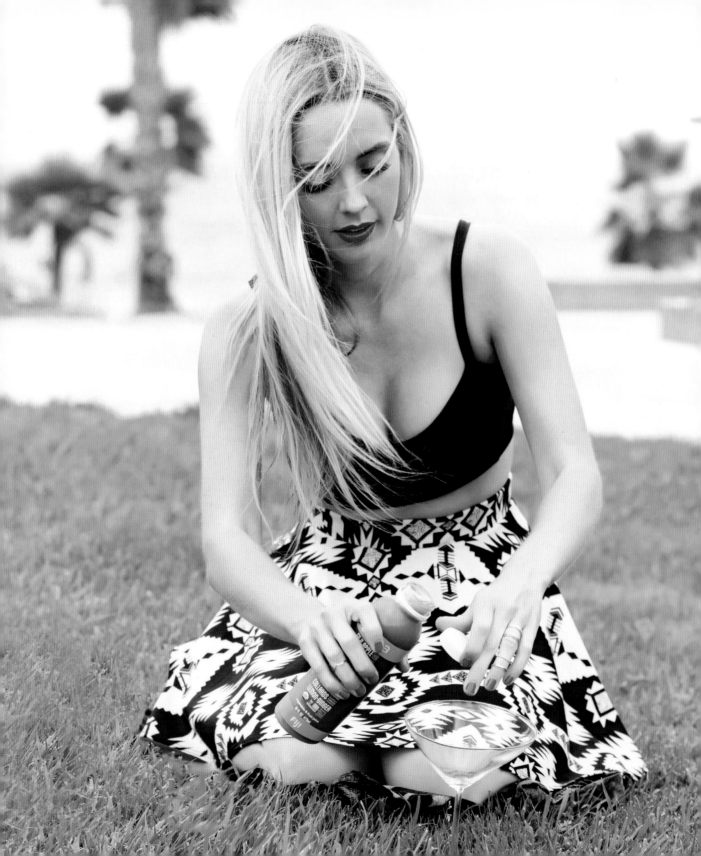

8

BUH-BYE, PIMPLES

LET'S START WITH MY FIVE SKIN CARE RULES:

+ You are what you freaking eat.
+ Don't overindulge in product.
+ Just because it works for your bestie, doesn't mean it will work for you.
+ The sun is aging you, so slather SPF on your face, neck and hands on the reg.
+ Keep it simple, stupid.

When people ask me about my skin care regime, I literally LOL.

It's so simple, it's almost embarrassing.

BUT WAIT.

Before I divulge my super-simple, easy, cheap tips, let me warn you: Just because my routine works swimmingly for me, doesn't mean it will work perfectly for everyone.

So that brings me to my first point:

YOU ARE WHAT YOU FREAKING EAT.

If you eat like shit, it will definitely come out on your skin.

Don't believe me?

Here's a little proof: Try a juice cleanse.

Your skin will pretty much never look better than what it looks like after a cleanse. That's because a cleanse flushes out all the nasty-ass toxins. After a juice detox, the skin is literally glowing like a pregnant woman's.

YUP, YUP, YUP.

Clear, radiant skin is one of the many benefits of cleansing.

Some of my suggestions for a clear complexion can be found at your local grocery store.

Check it:

Kale: Ahhhh, kale. This vegetable is The Shit. It's full of so many vits, like A, B, C, E and K. The gorgeous green is also full of iron, potassium, protein, phosphorus and manganese. Kale is number one on my list for a reason: It will make the complexion shine bright like a diamond. Some of my favorite ways to eat (or drink) kale include: homemade salads, fresh juices, kale chips and mixed with quinoa.

YUMMERS.

Blueberries: How amazing does a kale and blueberry salad sound? OK, just saying. Blueberries are the best natural antioxidant; they fight free radicals caused by ultraviolet (UV) radiation and sick-o pollution. Oh! Another benefit of these sexy berries? They're anti-aging. Blueberries can be thrown on top of Greek yogurt, blended into any type of smoothie and sprinkled over steel-cut oatmeal.

Salmon: This little fish heals cells, making them appear more youthful. Salmon's filled with omega fatty acids, which promote healthy, glowing skin. Add some lemon, chili flakes and ground pepper to it and you're set for a protein-filled dinner.

Nuts (unsalted): These babies will make/keep the skin plump and vibrant. It also doesn't hurt that nuts (almonds, especially) are filled with vitamin E. DIY trail mix by making a nut jar. Throw in dark chocolate chips, unsweetened coconut flakes and/or sunflower seeds. I also love adding nuts to anything I'm baking (brownies, cookies, cakes, etc.).

Flaxseeds: Poor, poor flaxseeds. They're often left in the dust. People know about them but tend to forget them. Well, neglect flaxseeds no longer, peeps, because they fight acne. Yes. This seed is known to take away inflammation. Eat up! Add them to oatmeal, Greek yogurt with fruit, baking recipes, smoothies or on top of salads.

Sweet potatoes: Oh, you know. Only my absolute favorite food ever. Like, ever, ever. People automatically give sweet potatoes a bad rap because they're in the potato family (which many associate with too many carbs). But hey—listen up! Sweet potatoes are king. Not only are they filled with vitamin A, but they also combat free radicals, which cause aging. Oh, and P.S. Vitamin A is the leading ingredient in many overpriced acne medications. I enjoy a sweet potato baked with a good organic, dairy-free butter, such as Earth Balance®.

Oranges: You've heard this since you were little: Oranges are packed with vitamin C. But wait. That doesn't mean go chug pasteurized orange juice. That actually means go eat (or juice it yourself) an organic orange. Foods like tomatoes, melons and oranges are filled with vit C, which helps protect the skin from scarring. So later, pock marks! Oranges to the rescue. My favorite way to eat an orange is in a salad. I mix berries, orange slices and kiwi together with four squeezes of lemon and a natural, herbal sweetener like Stevia. Add a sprinkle of cinnamon and thank me later.

Eggs: If a food could be my boyfriend, it would be eggs. I could eat them for breakfast, lunch and dinner. They're packed with protein, filled with antioxidants and contain lots of vitamin E. And! Eggs keep you full for hours. Total win. I prefer scrambled eggs with spicy mango salsa, egg salad with Dijon mustard or an old-fashioned hard-boiled egg with Himalyan pink salt and pepper.

IF YOU WANT TONS OF PIMPLES, EAT A TON OF THESE THESE JUNKY FOODS:

White bread: Unfortunately, white bread causes antinutrients (boo, boo!), meaning it's difficult for your bod to absorb any kind of nutrients, vitamins or minerals.

Salt: It's bloating and causes inflammation (hello, acne!).

Sugar: Tends to damage collagen and elastin.

Alcohol: It's one of the most dehydrating things you can consume.

If you want the best gas for your car, don't you want the best foods for your body and skin?

Remember: What you fuel your bod with in a decade will appear on your skin in the next; i.e., what you eat in your 30s will show on your skin in your 40s, and so on and on. Eat like shit = look like shit.

OK, so now that we're clear on what to eat and what not to eat for healthy skin, let's talk product.

DON'T OVERINDULGE IN PRODUCT.

I gotta admit, I enjoy a quiet chuckle when I see a girl with 50 pounds of skin-care product.

I mean, do they really think all that crap will magically transform their skin to rival J-Lo's?

(SIGH).

I'm going to share my biggest skin care secret: a bar of all-natural soap.

How stupidly, ridiculously easy is it to buy a bar of soap?

Let me tell you a little fairy tale. A long time ago a pimply princess went to a holistic skin doctor. The princess couldn't figure out what the hell was happening to her princess-y skin. The holistic skin doctor told her to stop all of her product use and buy an all-natural bar of soap to use twice a day. The pimply princess went home and tried the holistic skin doctor's recommendation. After a few days, the princess was no longer zitty—she was now a glowing, radiant princess (me)!

YOU HEARD IT HERE FIRST.

Go run (yes, run) to your local organic market and pick up a generic (let's not get crazy; there's no reason to buy Hawaiian, strawberry or coconut) bar of soap. Make sure it's all-natural and organic.

None of that chemical shit...'k?

It's not rocket science.

Wondering what to use for makeup remover?

Grape seed oil. It works like a charm and it's all-natural.

Oh, and need an amazing moisturizer? Grape seed oil works wonders! Just make sure you use an all-natural SPF afterward.

A toner?

Ya don't need it while you're experimenting with your all-natural bar of soap.

Makeup?

Keep it simple for the week you're doing the soap bar experiment.

And, obviously, practice the above healthful eating tips.

Try this tip for a week and see if it works for you.

For me, it was a real life changer.

Since then I've incorporated Cetaphil® into my routine a couple times a week. I love using the Clarisonic® cleansing systems once a week, too. Also, I try to get a facial every couple of months, use an all-natural SPF and make sure my face makeup is washed off before I go to sleep (again, grape seed oil is your new bestie for MU remover—throw away the chemical crap; it causes white dots under the eyes).

Moisturizing is key. I've found that organic products such as Eminence® (no, they're not paying me to say that) are amazing. They're filled with probiotics and contain all-natural ingredients (can you tell I like all-natural ingreds?).

A common mistake: Young girls using a Clarisonic-like tool every day or every other day. Um, hello! You're stripping your skin's natural collagen. Let the skin heal for a few days after exfoliating.

Exfoliating isn't meant to be practiced every day. In my opinion, if you're under 35, once a week is enough. If you're older than 35, two to three days a week is fine.

Simplify your skin care routine for better results. Everything doesn't have to be so complicated. Too many beauty products are a pain in the ass and usually overkill.

Which brings me to the next rule.

JUST BECAUSE IT WORKS FOR YOUR BESTIE, DOESN'T MEAN IT WILL WORK FOR YOU.

OMFG.

You know what's annoying?

When people think that just because something works for them, it will work for everyone.

Like, just because I'm obsessed with peaches, doesn't mean my dad is.

EVERYONE IS DIFFERENT.

And that applies to skin care, too.

You've lived with your body all your life. Use mind/body connection to figure out what skin care methods work best for you.

If you have oily-ass skin, stay away from oily-ass foundation.

If you have super dry skin, make sure to always take your makeup off, keep coffee consumption to once a day (drink more water, less coffee) and use a moisturizer that's all-natural (am I annoying you now?).

Oh, and dear Pimple Poppers: If you're going to mess with your skin, wash your freaking hands and use a tissue after a hot shower. Make sure you don't spread the pimple juice (I know, gross, right?) all over your face, because the pimple's juice is what causes zits to spread everywhere. Ever had one pimple that's turned into a small patch of pimples? You probably accidentally had the pimple juice spread. Yes, it's disgusting to talk about, but someone's got to do it. Love, me.

Anyway, back to rule number three. Be very careful when it comes to testing friends' products. The worst is when you're out shopping with friends and there are testers.

Testers scare me.

Experimentation is great (ESP when it's all-natural). But experiment smart.

Before you slather a lotion promising to cure wrinkles all over your pretty little face, test it on a tiny patch of skin.

EASY, PEASY.

The only thing that should be universally mandatory when it comes to skin care is chugging water. If you and your bestie want to copy one another when it comes to water, be my guest.

Everyone's skin is different. Do what works best for you, not your neighbor, not your grandma and not your dog . . . you!

THE SUN AGES YOU, SO SLATHER SPF ON YOUR FACE, NECK AND HANDS ON THE REG.

And then there's anti-aging.

Aging can be difficult. It's no fun looking in the mirror and seeing a number eleven between your eyes.

My take on anti-aging skin care is do what works for you. Again, my favorite anti-aging products are by Eminence Organic Skin Care. The products work well with my skin.

But ya wanna know my biggest anti-aging tips?

A hat and SPF.

I'm that dork who wears a hat every day. Hey! Incidental sun exposure, peeps!

If I'm running an errand, I throw on a hat.

(**Side note:** I might or might not have just purchased sun-protectant driving gloves. Yes. Driving gloves. They protect my hands from the sun!).

Sun is the devil.

LIKE, SO SORRY, "JERSEY SHORE"!

At least when it comes to the skin (this includes your hands, neck, arms, legs, feet, etc., not just your precious face).

I know what they say: "You need vitamin D."

There are other ways to get vitamin D besides basking in the sun like Magda from "There's Something About Mary."

Throw away your sick-ass sunning foil and smarten up.

Here are the facts that no one wants to hear: The link between tanning and skin cancer is cray, cray.

Even though there are studies everywhere to confirm this, women still lie in the sun without sunscreen.

When girls ask me about my skin, the first thing I say is: "SUNSCREEN and wear a freaking hat."

I know, I know. But you "look better with a tan (cry/whine/sigh)."

Welp, you don't look better with skin cancer cut out of your face. Or sunspots. Or pigmentation.

Instead of the sun, use the spray tan booth. It's easy and quick. Just make sure you exfoliate and shave before and moisturizer afterward. Also, wash the bottoms of your feet and your hands immediately after you're done in the booth.

Spray tanning has worked wonders for me. I do it about once every two weeks. The best part: absolutely NO UV rays!

Point: If you want flawless skin, keep it the hell out of the evil sun.

So, if you're trying to avoid pigmentation, freckles and sunspots on your skin (I'm guessing—hoping—this applies to everyone in the world?), then keep a hat, sunscreen and sunglasses in your oversized handbag.

KEEP IT SIMPLE, STUPID.

Stress comes out on your face.

Being stressed will make any pimple, zit or blackhead worse.

Don't overcomplicate life or skin care. Less stress will keep your skin clear and your life more manageable.

When people are stressed, a hormone called cortisol is released into the system. This mean, old hormone is a ruiner. It tries to ruin your skin's collagen and sleep patterns, and gets in the way of maintaining that sought-after six pack. Stress mostly robs the skin of important nutrients and creates less oxygen flow.

NO FUN.

Something that *can* benefit your skin is a mask. Here is my favorite all-natural, homemade mask:

THE SKINNY CONFIDENTIAL'S SEX KITTEN COCONUT MASK

1 tbsp/15 ml coconut oil
5 drops of apple cider vinegar
A few drops of lavender oil
½ tsp/1 g turmeric powder

+ Mix all together, rub on face and leave on for twenty minutes. Wash off with a warm towel. You can also use this mask on your arms and neck (don't forget about taking care of your neck; the skin is delicate and needs special attention!).

To sum it up: Skin care shouldn't be some super-crazy puzzle. In a nutshell: Drink lots of fresh veggie juices; consume fruits, vegetables, fish and eggs; chug water; don't be a certifiable product junkie; stay out of the sun; keep it simple; and, most importantly, do what works best for you!

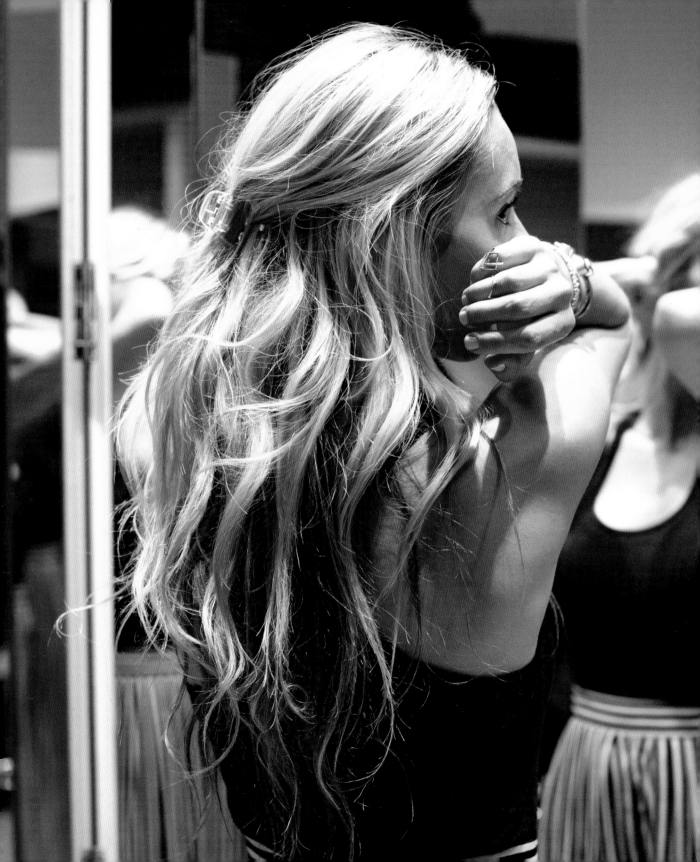

9

HAIR, HAIR
AND MORE HAIR

Whenever I'm having a great hair day, I feel like a girl from a Pantene Pro-V® commercial.

I smile bigger. My outfit doesn't seem to matter as much.

And overall, I just feel like I'm radiating more confidence.

Because let's face it: Hair is *muy importante.*

I'm going to provide the breakdown of one of my favorite topics: hair. It doesn't matter if yours is short, long, thick, curly, wavy, messy, dirty—we all have one thing in common: We all love good hair days.

I MEAN, RIGHT?

Let's start from the beginning:

Shampoo: My relationship with you is complicated. Sometimes I like it, sometimes I don't. I'm a big believer in shampooing (or washing hair, for that matter) only twice a week, sometimes once a week.

Before you stop reading this book because you're so disgusted, listen up.

If you wash your hair every day, you're doing two things: damaging your hair (ESP if it's colored) and wasting your time. Time that could be spent reading, relaxing or on more-productive activities.

I discovered that not washing my hair all the time made my hair shinier, thicker and more luscious.

Also, who doesn't love hippie chic hair? It's kinda cool if ya really think about it.

Long, natural, relaxed hair is making a comeback.

Overdone, beauty pageant hair is nasty.

Honestly, I can't believe it even had a moment.

OK. BACK TO SHAMPS.

I have many friends who have adopted the no-poo method. This is where they skip the shampoo altogether and go straight for the conditioner.

I've heard mixed reviews. For the no-poo method, I swear by products such as WEN® by Chaz Dean in Sweet Almond Mint or Fig Cleansing Conditioner. Most two-in-one conditioners strip the color out of the hair. Not this one. It cleanses and provides the right amount of moisture. Also, Wen® is awesome because it's free of sulfates and chemicals and contains absolutely no detergent. Some of my friends say they have to use Wen® only once a week! Sounds like heaven, right?

If you're into shampooing your hair, make sure you're using a paraben-free and sulfate-free brand. My favorite kind is by Moroccanoil®. It smells delish and works wonders on my rat's nest.

So. My main point in regard to shampoo is to use it sparingly. There's no reason to clean your hair every.single.day.

If you cut back on the washes, get ready for some serious dream hair.

Conditioner: Clearly conditioner is a must-have (ESP if you're doing the no-poo method).

Conditioner doesn't have to be just that white, creamy substance that everyone uses after shampoo. The right leave-in conditioner can rock your world. My preference is Biolage Daily Leave-In Tonic by Matrix®. I find if I don't use a leave-in conditioner, my hair is difficult to brush through and doesn't smell as yummy. So find one that works for you, and use it!

As far as using normal conditioner in the shower, don't let it touch the hair's root. If conditioner touches the roots, it tends to make the hair appear greasy and gross. I like to put conditioner only on the bottom half of my hair. Works like a charm!

Dry shampoo: Dry shampoo is a powder-like shampoo that doesn't need to be washed out with water. I throw it in my gym bag because it takes one second to apply and is great for ridding the hair of sweat or grease. It's perfect for when you don't have time to wash your hair. If you're out of dry shamps, use baby powder. It has the same effects and makes dirty hair appear clean. Dry shampoo is especially effective after a workout (hint, hint).

Brushes: They're everything. If you own a shitty brush, be prepared for crazy hair.

I literally could not live without my Wet Brush™.

IT'S A LIFE CHANGER.

I'm not big into brushing my hair, so I use the Wet Brush™. A Wet Brush™ is a hairbrush that works really well for ridding the hair of knots. It's the only brush I've found that doesn't pull on my hair or hurt my scalp. It's very hair-friendly. And does wonders for my rat's nest.

I've never been one of those girls like Marcia Brady who counts her brush stokes, but let me tell ya: The Wet Brush™ gets the job done.

Especially (and obviously) when the hair is wet. Instead of sweating from hair brush frustration and spending an extra twenty minutes brushing your locks, you'll spend about a minute.

Blow dryers, straighteners, curling irons, etc.: I honestly cringe when people tell me they blow dry, straighten and/or curl their hair on the reg. Hair needs a break. I will put heat on my hair once a week at most. If you ever see someone whose hair is fried, it's typically the result of one of two things: a bad hair extension job or overuse of hair dye and/or heat. Keep the heat away from your head as much as possible. Also, if you're using a blow dryer, make sure it's an ionic blow dryer. They're known to promise twice the water removal, which means there's less heat damage. I know no one wants to hear this, but straight irons are worse than blow dryers. And please, oh please, stay away from blow dryers with 400°F/200°C settings unless you're working with a professional. I mean, you're practically ironing your hair. Kinda nasty when you think about it, huh? Make sure you're always using the lowest setting possible. To add extra protection, work as quickly as possible.

My biggest hair tip when it comes to heat: Let your hair air dry for as long as possible before you use heated tools!

Rollers: Call me old school, but I love a good drugstore roller. They're cheap and easy to use. I throw them in my hair (starting front to back) while I'm doing my makeup all the time. I only use them on the middle part of my hair, though; I keep the sides of the hair down. Rollers provide some body and make the hair appear clean (even if it's dirty and gross—lol).

DIY beach waves: Who doesn't love beach waves?! They're effortlessly chic and so, so easy. Make your own DIY beach wave spray using an empty spray bottle. Use a tablespoon/15 g of sea salt (per 8 oz/240 ml of water), ½ teaspoon/2 ml of coconut oil, two to five drops of tea tree oil and one dab of all-natural hair gel. Use the DIY spray on damp or dry hair. And *voilà!* You've got yourself some sexy, bombshell waves.

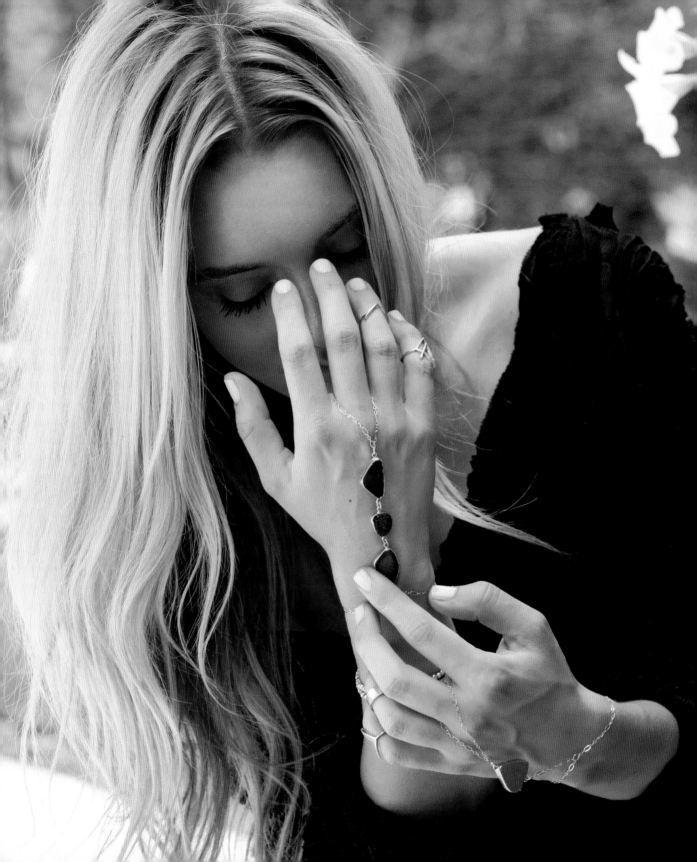

The hippie chic look: Ahhhh. My favorite look. Typically in pictures, this is the look I always go for. So WTF is hippie chic hair? Welp, it's the "I don't give an F" look. Too cool for school, rock 'n' roll, sex kitten look. My trick for hippie chic hair (don't laugh): Assuming I want this look for a Saturday, I'll curl my hair outward (but super, super tight) on Friday afternoon.

Side note: I'm obviously not venturing out into civilization on Friday night because I absolutely despise that tight-curled, pageant look. I spray my hair and sleep on it. Yes, I sleep on it. Sleeping on it allows the curls to completely relax. When I wake up, I shake it out again and then put it in a low, low (like at the nape of the neck) bun and clip it with a tiny alligator clip. Then I spray the bun once with a bit of hair spray. I go about my day with a low bun. By Saturday night, I shake it out again and add a tiny bit more spray (I love, love, love Dove® Extra Hold travel-size hair spray; it's light and it smells yummy). And I'm ready to par-tay. Here's the cool thing about this look: Sometimes my hair will look even better by Sunday! This is totally amazing for someone who hates heat damage.

The Victoria's Secret curl: Here's the trick to how those gorgeous girls get their hair looking so amaze: Curl outward. Sound easy? It's not. After you've washed your hair, let it air dry for about twenty minutes. Then, using a blow dryer (on a low setting, of course), dry your hair straight. Grab a heated curling iron and make sure the iron is parallel to your face as you curl downward and outward. Use an alligator clip to do your hair in sections. When you curl the hair, make sure you leave a 1-inch/25-mm section sticking out at the end. That will provide those long, long, beautiful curls. The most important part: Make sure the pieces in front of your face are really curled outward. Spray hair with a light hair spray and shake out the curls a bit. You want it to look like you didn't spend hours on your hair, so the shake is essential. Oh, and FYI: If you want to look like Shirley Temple or attain bridal hair (<< opposite of VS hair), then position the curling iron perpendicular and curl inward.

Post-pool hair: If I had my way, I would wear a swimming cap every time I swam. But I don't really think that look's in right now. A quick, easy trick for the pool is to precondition your hair. Applying conditioner before going into the pool helps to protect the hair from nasty-ass chlorine damage. And obviously: Wash your hair as soon as possible when you're done swimming. Also!!! NEVER go into the pool with a braid; it will break your hair.

Split ends: Call me crazy, but I love the split-end look. When people ask me why my hair is so long, I tell them my dirty, little secret: I cut it once a year (if that), and when I don't cut it, I get it "dusted." Uhhh...I know what you're thinking: "WTF is dusting?" Dusting is a technique where the stylist doesn't take any length off; she just carefully snips the split ends off. The hair that's taken off is so fine that it looks just like dust on the ground. Love, die, dead. My favorite trick on earth.

In any case, I feel like hairdressers all had a secret meeting and decided that if they told the world that their hair wouldn't grow unless it was cut every three months, then they would make more money. I'm living proof that if you don't cut your hair frequently, it will grow as long as you want. Besides, split ends are kind of "in" right now. That hippie chic Lauren Conrad look is hot, hot, hot. Dust away, ladies!

Hairstylist tips: Pick a stylist who has amazing hair. I think it's weird when people go to hairdressers who have crappy hair. I mean, would you go to a doctor who was obese and sick? Probs not. So pick someone who has beautiful hair and knows what the hell he or she is doing.

Color: If you are like me, you color your hair. Please, please, please use a shampoo and conditioner that protects the color. ESP if you've spent an arm and leg on color, you want to preserve your color, not ruin it! Also, if you're blonde, purple shampoo is a game changer; it takes the brassiness out of the hair and brightens the highlights.

Hair sunscreen: I use hair sunscreen just as much as I use regular SPF. Why? Well, because hair is also affected by the sun's rays. My favorite is by Biolage and it's known to shield the hair from UV rays. Use this daily and use extra for pool days.

OK, LET'S DISCUSS THE NITTY-GRITTY.

When it comes to your luscious locks, staying away from parabens and sulfates is a must.

But why?

Because they're nasty-ass chemicals that you don't want anywhere near your precious scalp. And if you can avoid them, why not?

They have the potential to cause skin irritation, eye irritation and damage to the hair follicles. Parabens, specifically, act as a preservative that supposedly rids bacteria.

Cheers to shiny, pretty hair!

Keep that crap away from your skin and hair; trust me.

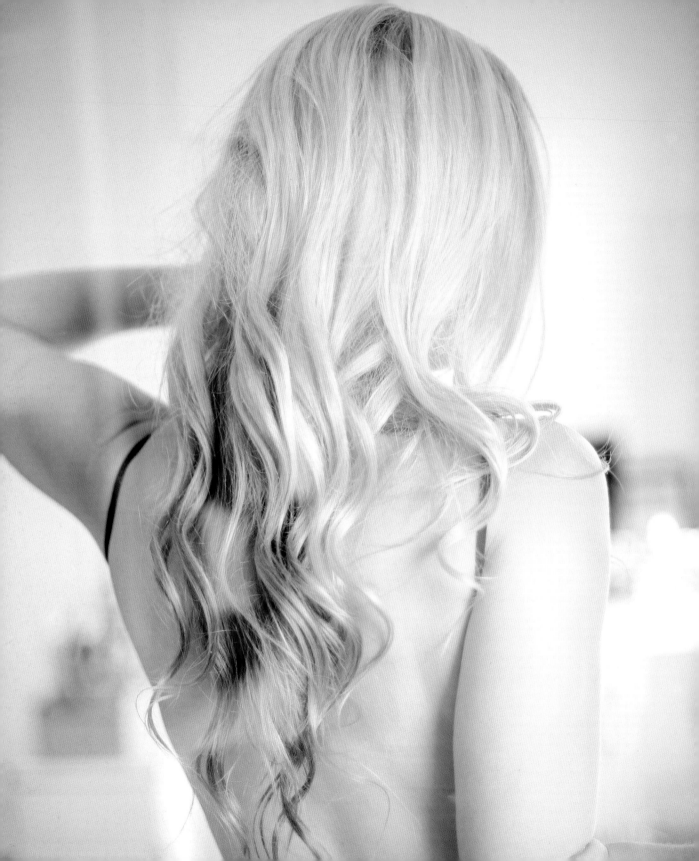

Side note: Try to check all your products for sulfates and parabens. These suckers hide in moisturizers, makeup products and toothpaste.

Obviously you can't control every product you use, but if you have the opportunity to choose, why not choose wisely?

And please oh please, eat your hair vitamins. There are so many foods that will promote hair growth and shine. Some of my favorite hair foods are: spinach, oysters, salmon, nuts, lentils and blueberries.

Check out my favorite hair care smoothie.

Overall, I eat these foods as much as possible, because who doesn't like long, healthy hair?!

I'm also a big fan of massaging my scalp while showering. A deep massage on the scalp is known to promote hair growth and increase circulation. It's also an amazing way to de-stress.

Oh, and naturally; my boyfriend gets a massage from me on his scalp daily—balding prevention!!

So! There you have it, all my sex kitten, dirty hair tricks/tips.

THE SKINNY CONFIDENTIAL'S BOMBSHELL HAIR CARE CONCOCTION

1 handful of spinach
2 handfuls of organic blueberries
3 splashes of raw coconut water
1 tbsp/10 g flaxseeds
1 tbsp/10 g chia seeds

+ Blend together with a handful of ice.

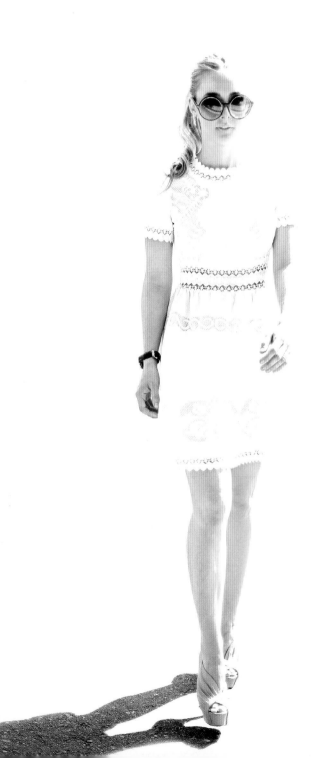

10

FLATTER
YOUR BOD

Fact: Just because it looked good on Rihanna doesn't mean it will look good on you.

And, hey! Something else might look amazing on you and horrible on Rihanna!

Kim Kardashian is someone who is guilty of following trends. She simply doesn't dress for her body type.

Like, sorry, Kanye; you're not picking the right style for Kimmy K. **TRY AGAIN.**

My advice? Don't follow the trends if they don't work for you. Super white, tight jeans just don't flatter everyone.

Get over it because there are 6 million other pairs of pants that will make your butt look insane.

Typically, women fall into four categories: circle (thick around the waist); triangle (a bigger bottom half); hourglass (curvy but pretty much proportioned); and rectangle (straight up and down).

The Circle: Choose tops that are baggy around the waist. Try to avoid clothing like high-waisted pants and bell-bottoms. Belts are your worst enemy. Go for tunics and skinny jeans.

The Triangle (this is Kim's shape): Don't go for oversized shirts or sweaters, skinnies and/or silk fabrics. A black pair of wide-leg jeans will slim the thighs and create a long, lean look.

The Hourglass: Avoid boxy shirts, tunics and oversized shirts. Go for high-waisted jeans. It will draw people's eye to your skinny midsection! And you can't go wrong with V-neck tops.

The Rectangle: You want to buy styles that hug the waistline and flare out at the bottom. Boot-cut jeans/pants are your bestie. A fitted blazer also will slim the waist instantly.

Just because something looks great on someone else, don't automatically assume you have-to-have-it-or-you'll-die-because-it's-so-so-cute.

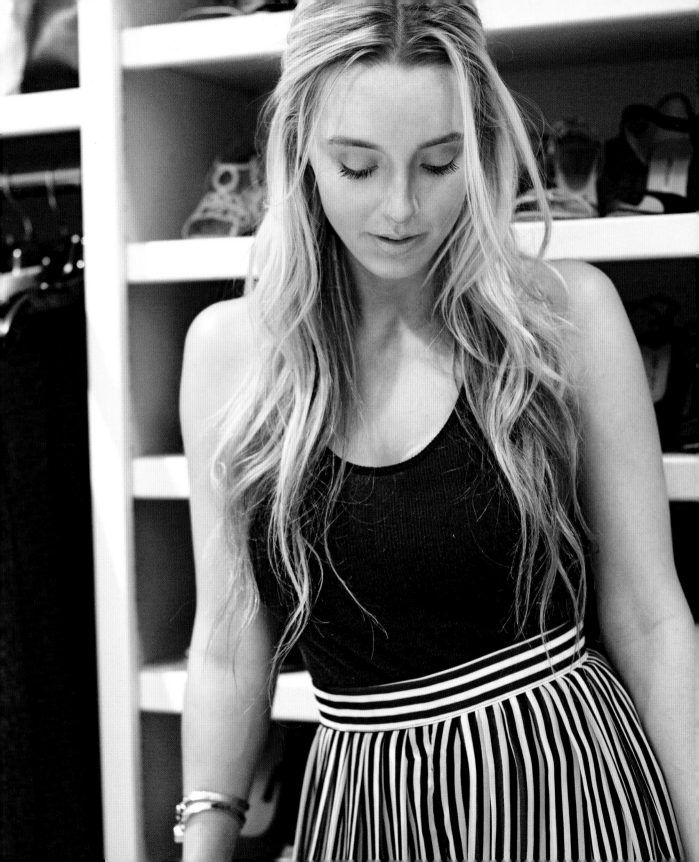

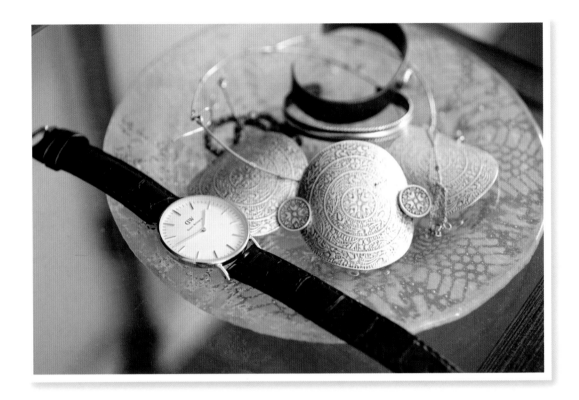

I love purchasing lots of blacks (think skinny jeans, long-sleeved sweaters, oversized tops—all in black). They're obvious staples and work well with any splash of color.

Also, altering is like God's gift to fashion.

I talk to my seamstress more than I talk to my boyfriend.

Any great seamstress can fix any outfit. Getting clothes tailored to your body is a game changer.

If a seamstress isn't in the budget, just make sure you're choosing clothing that works well for you.

Not your friend, not your neighbor, not your favorite celeb—YOU.

I'd love to wear white pants on the reg, but they aren't flattering on me. I hate how they make my ass look.

If you're on your period and your bloat is seriously out of control, adopt the "homeless chic" look.

The homeless chic look was created by MK and Ashley Olsen. It's where you adorn yourself in the baggiest clothes possible but still look cute.

I like to steal my boyfriend's clothes when "Aunt Flow" is in town. Normally, she brings along an extra 5 pounds/2 kg, so I plan accordingly. I die over his flannels, collared shirts and vintage tees. I tuck them into my skinny jeans with boots and I'm good to go. Add a long chain and a super-cute hat for extra detail.

Stealing boys' sunglasses/hats/watches is always fun, too! I mean, you don't want to look like a baggy hobo, so keep it sexy. Tucking shirts into jeans and adding a few feminine touches to men's clothes is hot!

My boyfriend's clothes allow me to achieve that effortless, homeless-chic look, while dressing for my menstrual cycle.

FUN TIMES.

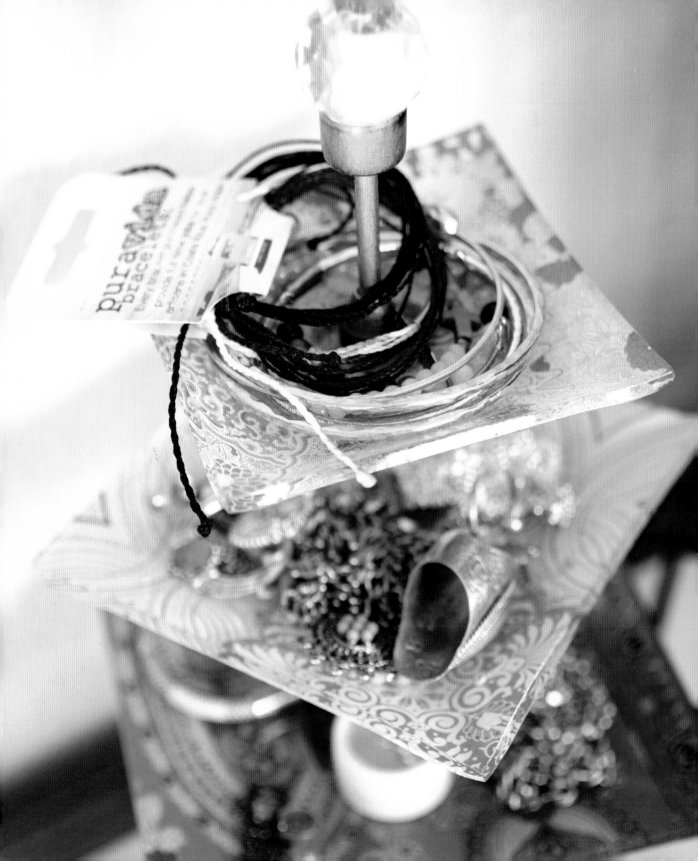

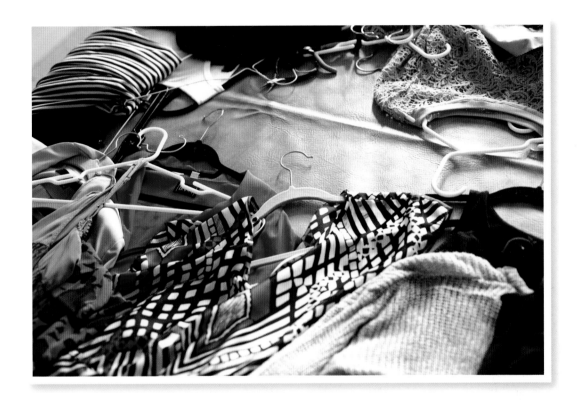

Anyway, my advice for anyone's wardrobe: Buy staples.

Some of my favies include:
+ A great pair of fitted jeans
+ Black skinny pants
+ An oversized, sexy cardigan
+ White pumps/heels
+ Black ankle boots
+ A white, short-sleeved tee
+ A draped black skirt (I prefer asymmetrical)
+ A maxi dress (opt for darker colors and make sure the dress is super long)

Accessory staples:

+ A long, thin, gold necklace

+ Tiny gold or silver stud earrings

+ A few thin rings

+ Big, huge hoops

+ A dainty handpiece

+ A coin purse with a long chain

+ A big, huge, absolutely absurdly large purse (I like white or black)

After you buy staples, you can plan around them. Some of my favorite stores that are chic and affordable include: Forever 21 (best finds ever; ya just have to search like you're looking for a needle in a haystack); Charlotte Russe; LuLu*s online, Target (cute little boot selection); Marshalls; Nasty Gal; and vintage stores.

Find your own style to reflect who you are. Many years ago, I was dressing like Barbie® on steroids. It just wasn't me and wasn't comfortable.

SO MALIBU BARBIE® HAD TO GO.

Since then, my whole closet has evolved. I like darker colors and whites. I own lots of ankle boots, rocker tees, flea market finds, maxi skirts and dresses, skinny jeans, off the shoulder sweaters, kimonos and jumpsuits.

I feel so much more comfortable now that I've found my style niche.

And hey, if you're looking good on the outside, make sure you're feeling good on the inside. There's nothing sexier than a confident, positive woman dressed to kill.

The more confidence you have, the better. Remember? Fake it, until you make it, peeps! Hopefully, by the time you finish this book, you'll be able to wear a paper bag and freaking own it.

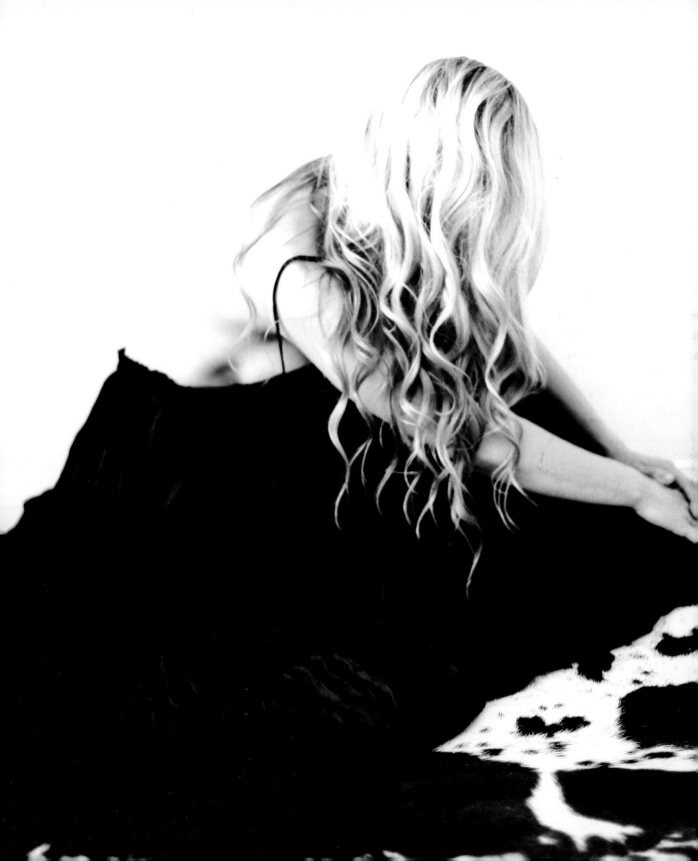

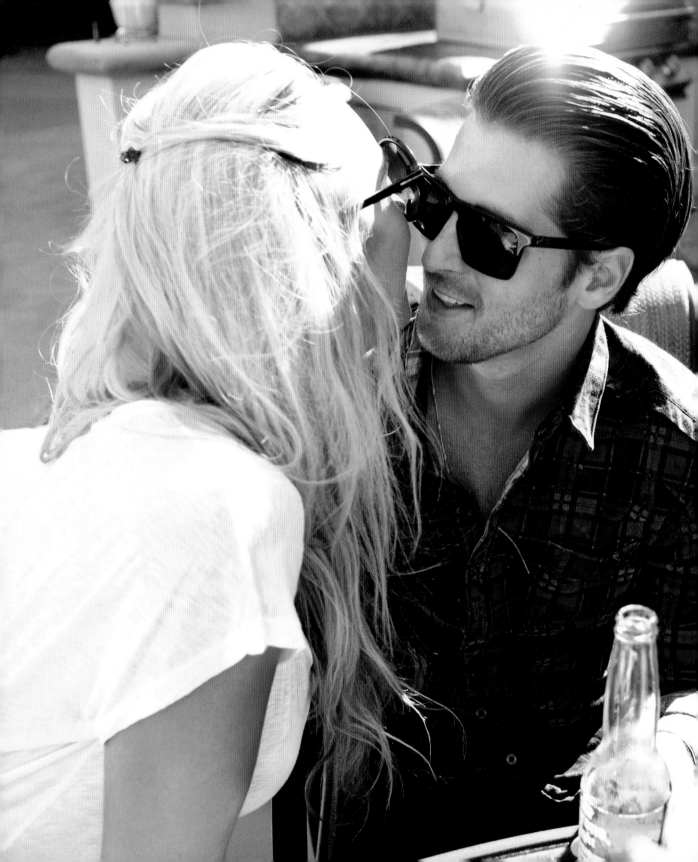

11

LOVE
CHUB

OK, so here's the deal: You meet a man (swoon!). You and Mr. Man fall deeply in love. Everything's hearts and freaking butterflies.

There's only one problem: His eating habits are absolutely horrendous.

He eats pizza, chips, white bread and sick crap all day long. But wait, you're so in love, so naturally you start to adopt his lovely habits.

This, my friends, is love chub.

And it's a total epic **FAIL.**

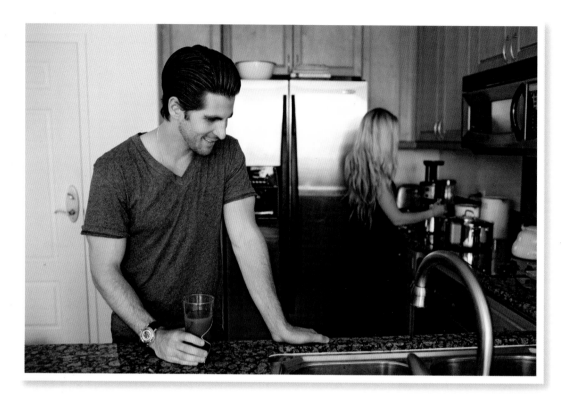

I've spoken with so many women who fall madly in love and start to eat like shit because of their BF's habits. Letting another person dictate your eating is about as ridiculous as picking up smoking because your partner puffs a pack a day.

Separate the relationship and the food.

It's a lot easier than you think, peeps.

My first trick is maybe somewhat manipulative (sorry, hunny!). I decided that instead of my babe influencing my eating, I'd influence his. Muhaha!

SO I BOUGHT A JUICER.

And every morning I juiced my little heart out. At first he walked by, curious. Later that week there were questions. Then, he requested a taste.

Guess what? Now he's practically a juicer connoisseur! He wakes me every A.M. with a cup of green juice. This is "healthy manipulation" at its finest, people.

Juicing together each morning is romantic, healthy and delicious (a total win/win).

HERE ARE A FEW RECIPES THAT WILL STEAL YOUR MAN'S HEART.

*Each juice fills a 16-ounce/450-ml cup

NOTE: Apples should NOT be blended or juiced with their seeds; they contain cyano compounds, which are carcinogenic in high enough amounts.

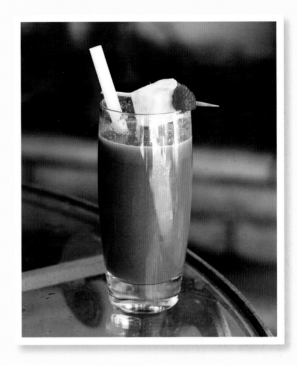

THE HEALTHY BLOODY MARY: A HANGOVER CURE

This is the perfect juice for Sundays. If your man's Saturday was rough, whip this hangover remedy up and enjoy in bed. Because, I mean, who doesn't love bloodies?! Cheers!

1 tomato
2 celery sticks
1 handful of spinach
1 lemon, squeezed
A few pinches of cayenne

+ Juice everything together

MR. MAN JUICE

This is one of my favorite juices because it helps with energy levels, aids in digestion and promotes healthy skin. It tastes similar to lemonade, too

2 handfuls of arugula

A handful of kale

1 green apple

1 lemon, squeezed

½ cucumber

½ ginger root, diced and peeled

+ Juice everything together

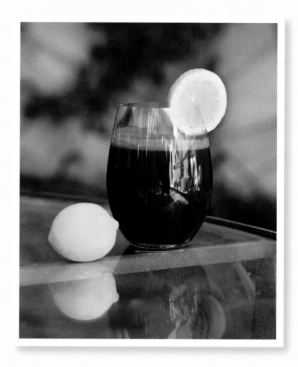

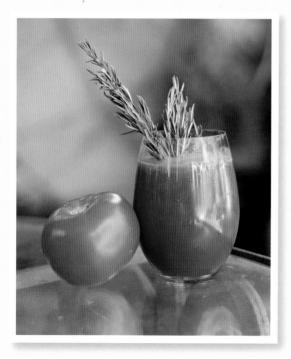

THE MEOW

This fresh juice is the most amazing anti-inflammatory. Cilantro and turmeric will whip out any inflammation. All the rest of the ingreds are filled with important vitamins and minerals. Beets are also fab for reducing blood pressure. This baby is definitely the most "veggish" and daring of the three. First-time juicers should try the first two before trying The Meow.

1 gala apple

A handful of beets

½ red bell pepper

1 large carrot

1 ginger root, diced and peeled

4 cilantro leaves

A few pinches of turmeric

+ Juice everything together

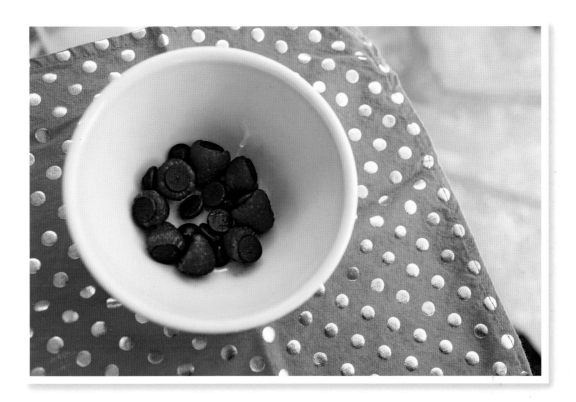

So let's talk fruit. Living with a significant other can be a real uphill battle (that's a whole separate book), but staying healthy as a couple is easy-peasy. Keep a bowl of organic apples, a stocked banana holder and some containers filled with berries on the kitchen counter. Fruit is high in enzymes, fiber, amino acids and vitamins. The more accessible the fruit, the better. Oh! And it satisfies a sweet tooth, too.

TOTALLY ROMANTIC, RIGHT?

Incorporate fruit into your and your partner's meals. Some examples: berries in oatmeal, watermelon slices in an arugula salad, cherries diced over chicken and bananas dipped in almond butter. Movie theater date? Pack some fresh raspberries stuffed with chocolate chips for you and your hunny to snack on.

Your taste buds and your ass will thank you later. Meanwhile, your boyfriend will start to see that white bread and pizza are not the only food groups on the planet.

SHOCKER!

Other foods that will rock your man's world: hummus, lentils, sweet potatoes, quinoa and veggie burgers.

OK, so eating out as a couple is a total relationship perk.

But hey, just because the BF orders fried calamari as an app, a steak dripping in butter with a side of French fries as an entree and a slice of cobbler for dessert doesn't mean you should, too. When I'm at a restaurant, I pay absolutely no attention to what anyone else is ordering. My favorite dining out tip: Say no to entrees. I usually choose a salad as an appetizer and then pick an appetizer in place of an entree. Substituting apps for entrees is an effective way to practice portion control.

I mean, it's not rocket science. If your partner orders eggs Benedict, is it necessary for you to order it, too? Absolutely not. Why? Because most likely, you're going to steal a few bites of his hollandaise-covered eggs anyway. Order yourself something light like scrambled eggs and a side of fruit; that way, a few bites of his order are no big deal. Having a boyfriend around really works to a healthy girl's advantage: They tend to order the decadent foods, making it easy for you to make guilt-free choices. You'll enjoy your meal with the option to steal a few bites of his. I call these "taste tests." Utilizing a partner for a taste test works like a charm. Instead of feeling deprived, have a taste test (this equals a few bites), and move on with your life.

Are you totally into exercise? While you're exercising, does your partner lie on the couch like a fat, lazy slob? Sound familiar? Please, oh, please do *not* change up your regular work-out routine because of your boyfriend, girlfriend, friend, dad, mom, neighbor, etc.
Your sweat sesh should always be about you.

But it never hurts to play the invite card.

I present the invitation: "Hunny? Yoga at noon?" If he goes, great. If he declines, not my problem. If you're with someone who isn't into working out, don't let his or her mindset dictate your exercise regime. I find exercising extremely therapeutic, and if I don't get my therapy, I'm a real bitch. No one wants to date a bitch; therefore, working out makes me a better partner. If your man loves to work out, then do it together. Take hikes, walk the dog, play tennis, join the same gym or ride bikes! Research shows that couples who work out together, stay together. Sweating together will improve your sex life, create a healthy competition and promote positive vibes.

SOME EXAMPLES OF COUPLE-FRIENDLY, AT-HOME EXERCISES:

P90X®: This workout video is available online. Pop this baby into the DVD player and sweat for an hour a day with your partner. Don't have one? Grab a friend.

Strength training: This is one of the most effective workouts! Think a half hour of on-the-floor abs, lunges, squats and arm workouts with 5-pound to 10-pound/2- to 5-kg weights (Don't have weights at home? Substitute water bottles), running in place or bicycle sit-ups. Use the Nike® app if you want more direction. I'm obsessed with the Nike® app because it personalizes each workout. For instance, the app's choices are: get lean, get toned, get strong or get focused. Your man can choose a customized "strong workout" while you sweat next to him with the "get lean workout." It's like having a personal trainer (there are about a hundred different workouts available) anywhere, anytime.

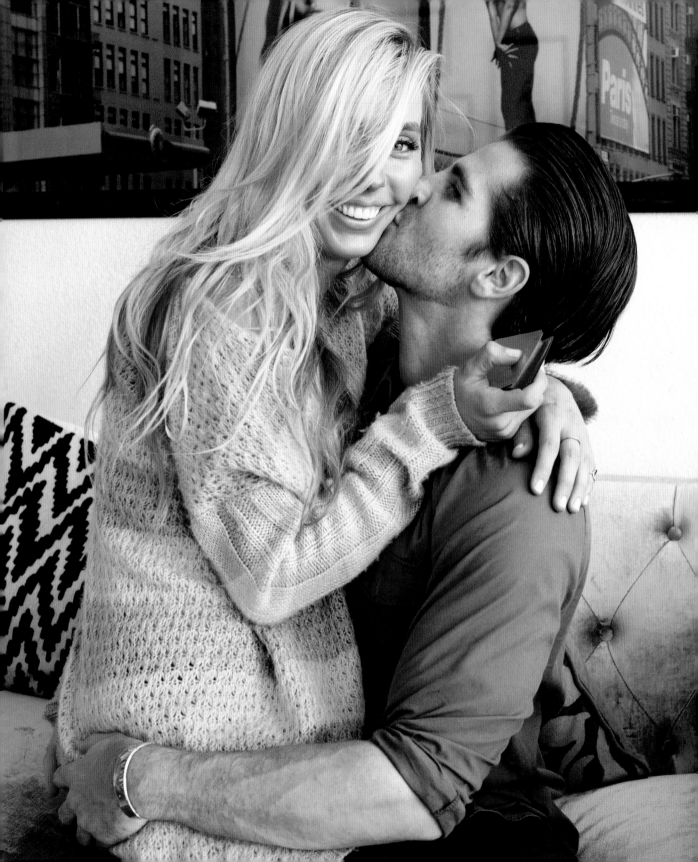

COOL? DUH.

Boxing: Pick up some gloves at the nearest Target and spar off with a partner. This work-out keeps the heart rate up and strengthens the upper body. Maintain a lunging position to work the legs.

Pilates and yoga: Hello, YouTube! Make use of the Internet; there's free access to a ton of Pilates and yoga workouts. Grab two yoga mats with your man and try de-stressing with light stretching and these Zen-like exercises. For an extra challenge, add push-ups, a few planks and tricep dips.

Sex: Ya. I went there. Sex = major calorie burning. Plus, it's fun.

And honestly, if your boy doesn't want to participate in healthy choices, then his loss. Besides, sometimes it's more fun to sweat by yourself anyway. You'll get time to yourself to focus on your own goals. Sucks for him!

Most importantly, be a role model for your partner. Eat clean, drink lots of water and sweat. Sooner or later he'll catch on to a healthy lifestyle.

See? There's absolutely no excuse for love chub!

So repeat after me: Just because your boy toy eats like shit, doesn't mean you eat like shit!

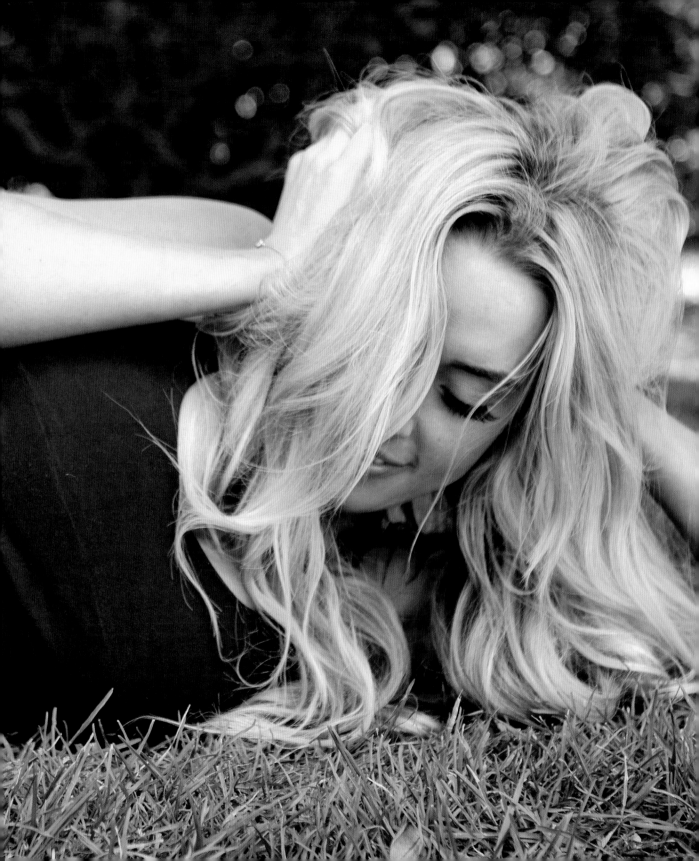

12

LEARN IT,
LIVE IT, LOVE IT

No excuses.

Today's the day.

The day to make some small changes that will have positive effects on the rest of your life.

From here on out, you're setting the tone for **YOUR** life. No one can do it for you.

Use your newfound confidence to create a healthy, happy life for yourself, your family and/or your friends.

When it comes to eating, make a commitment to know what's in your food.

Don't eat something out of habit or because you're sad or happy or bored. Eat it because it's beneficial to your health or it's delicious. If you're craving a slice of cake, have a slice and move on. Stop making food such a big deal.

Eat to live, don't live to eat.

If I can leave you with one food tip, it's this: If you're going to make the decision to put something with no nutrition into your mouth, then at least add nutrients to it.

EXAMPLES?

If you're eating a slice of pizza, add arugula, red onion, jalapeño slices and/or avocado.

If you're drinking coffee, add a good fat like all-natural, organic coconut milk, instead of sick-ass creamer.

If you're drinking alcohol, keep the added ingredients fresh (lemon, lime and blood orange cocktail, anyone?).

If you're eating cake, include a hefty side of berries.

After a while, you'll see that processed food really isn't that cool.

That routine cup of pasteurized orange juice doesn't taste as delicious as a cup of fresh-pressed green juice.

And maybe that bag of chips isn't as satisfying as a delicious baked sweet potato.

Forget about sick-o, store-bought sauces and dressings and start making your own. Get interested in what you're fueling your body with because the cold, hard truth is NO ONE is going to do it for you.

And when it comes to beauty, you're probably not always going to be able to find organic makeup and hair products, but if it's available, use it.

Rock your outfits—don't let them rock you.

Try to minimize your exposure to chemicals and nasty additives. And use SPF on the reg.

LITTLE CHANGES GO A LONG WAY.

Lastly, make an effort to sweat once a day (hey, sex counts!). Get your heart rate up and let those endorphins fly through your body. If you can get your partner to join you, you're a star. Live a healthy, happy life.

Because at the end of the day, life's about balance.

Balance is sustainable.

Balance is sexy.

Balance is a lifestyle.

Learn it. Live it. Love it.

xx,

>ACKNOWLEDGMENTS

I would like to thank my dad, Brad, for bringing out my entrepreneurial spirit. You've always believed in me and I love you so much!

I want to thank my stepmom, Julie, for constantly keeping me inspired. I'm so lucky to have you in my life. Also, my sisters, Faye and Mimi, and my brother, Myles, for always making me laugh—like really, really LOL. Thanks for keeping family dinners entertaining.

To an amazing mom, who always created the most beautiful, healthful, organic meals. Thank you for teaching me how to modify foods!

To my Nanz (AKA my sexy grandma), Mary Evarts, thank you for being my bestie. You're my absolute favorite.

A gazillion thanks to my godparents, Michael Bell (a kitchen guru!) and Jennifer Bell, who have become an extension of my family. You've been amazing role models, especially when it comes to healthy living. Love you both. Thaaannnkkkk you!

To the four people who helped to guide me every step of the way: my publisher, William Kiester; project editor, Marissa Giambelluca; designer, Meg Baskis; and literary agent, Marilyn Allen. I could not have done any of this without you four.

Huge thank you to Basil Vargas. Your photography gave the book color and life. And to a fantastic copy editor, Carol Terman Polakowski.

And thanks to Thomas Fitzsimmons, the best mentor for writing a book. Without you, I'd be screwed! Seriously, though!

I'm forever grateful to: Chris Keach (the webmaster!); Gary and Lisa Bosstick (both of you are always so supportive); and the Vogts, the Buells, and the Samays (love all of you!).

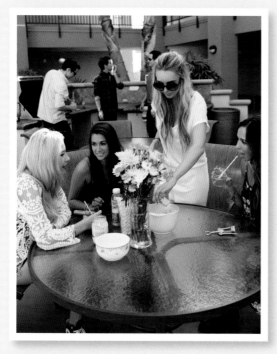

To all my sex kitten super babes—Briana, Lauren, Jackie, Tara, Jordan, Carly, Jacqueline, Stefanie, Tina, Annie, Elena, Rachel, Westin, Mark, Stephen, Dante, Rocco, Jeff, Farley and Ian—MWAH! You all kick ass.

To an insane business partner, Erica, who's helped make our blogging consulting biz a well-oiled machine. Love, love, love you!

To Steve Houck: You've believed in me since the second I meet you. Thank you for understanding my humor and totally "getting me." Your well-prepared PowerPoint presentation two years ago on The Skinny Confidential's brand has kept me focused and inspired. You're a life-long friend and I love you!

To my trainer, Mike, who makes sure there's no cheese on my ass!

Thank you times a mil to the readers of The Skinny Confidential, who continue to make blogging super F-ing fun.

And, of course, to my hearts, and the true loves of my life: the handsome Michael Bosstick and the most gorgeous Chihuahua in the world, Pixy Bean, who's definitely the best "spooner" ever.

>ABOUT THE AUTHOR

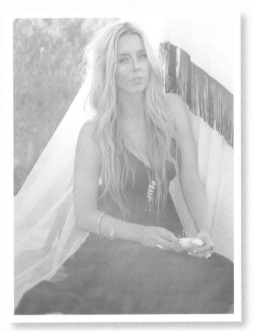

LAURYN EVARTS is the creator of the blog & brand The Skinny Confidential, which was named the top health/fitness blog in the world by Bloglovin'. Lauryn has worked with Free People, ViX swimwear, Benefit Cosmetics, Lionsgate Television and Victoria's Secret. She lives in San Diego, where she loves cooking, entertaining and spooning her Chihuahua, Pixy.

>INDEX

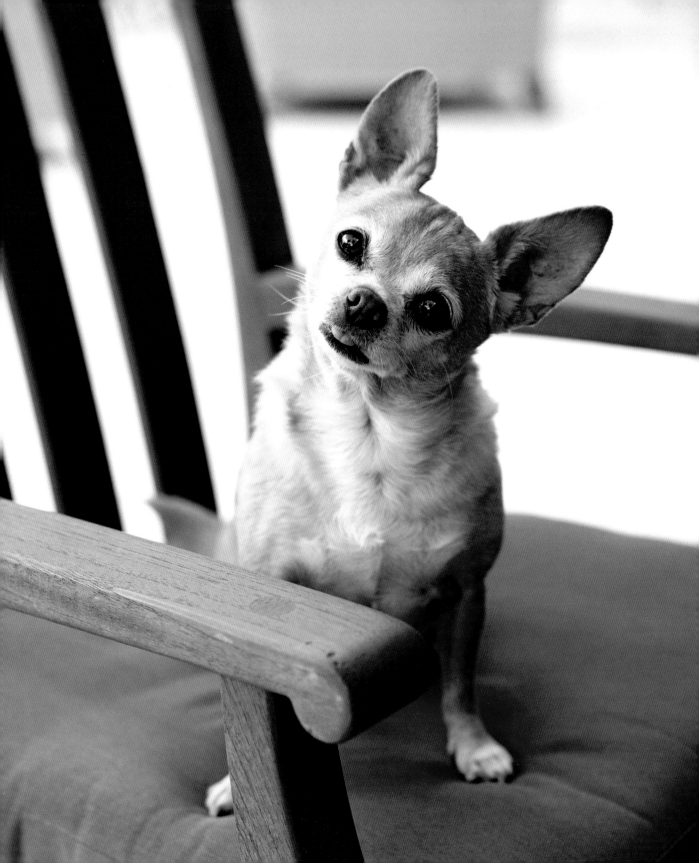